Change the Food, Change the World

Change the Food, Change the World

A Catholic Perspective on Fostering a Culture of Life Through a Plant-Based Diet

Paula Sandin and Jennifer Sandin Adams

Scripture quotations are from the *St. Joseph Edition of The New American Bible Revised Edition,* copyright © 2011 by the Catholic Book Publishing Corp., N.J. Used with permission.

Excerpts from the English translation of the *Catechism of the Catholic Church* for the United States of America copyright © 1994, United States Catholic Conference, Inc. - Libreria Editrice Vaticana. English translation of the *Catechism of the Catholic Church: Modifications from the Editio Typica* copyright © 1997, United States Catholic Conference, Inc. - Libreria Editrice Vaticana. Used with permission.

Change the Food, Change the World™ is a trademark of A Litttle Light, LLC.

© 2018 Paula Sandin and Jennifer Sandin Adams
All rights reserved.

ISBN-13: **9781986340946**
ISBN-10: **1986340945**

This book is not intended as a substitute for the medical advice of doctors. The reader should regularly consult a physician in matters relating to his/her health particularly with respect to any symptoms that may require medical attention, diagnosis, or treatment. Persons choosing to adopt the food choices discussed in the book should first consult a physician before making any dietary changes. Food can serve as a powerful agent such that medications may need to be adjusted in just a few days' time. This should be taken very seriously. The publisher and authors accept no liability should readers adopt the dietary suggestions made in this book. Mention of specific organizations or authorities does not imply that they endorse this book, its authors, or the publisher. References are provided for informational purposes only and do not constitute endorsement of any websites or other sources. Readers should be aware that the websites listed in this book may change.

Contents

To Our Readers · IX

Foreword · XI

Open Letter to Pope Francis · · · · · · · · · · · · · · · · XV

Introduction · XXI

Part I: Life Seeds · 1

Chapter 1   Human Health · 3

Chapter 2   Reproduction and Hormones · · · · · · · · · · · · · · · 25

Chapter 3   The Poor and the Hungry · · · · · · · · · · · · · · · · · 35

Chapter 4   The Environment · 43

Chapter 5   Animals · 51

Part II: Our Response · 61

Chapter 6 Bridging the Political Divide · · · · · · · · · · · · · · · · · · 63

Chapter 7 The Church's Role · 71

Chapter 8 Change the Food, Change the World · · · · · · · · · · · 74

Part III: Common Objections · 79

Chapter 9 Common Objections and Our Responses · · · · · · · · 81

          About The Authors · 97

          Our Favorite Resources · 99

          References · 103

To Our Readers...

We are very grateful Catholic converts. Our book was written through the lens of our treasured Catholic faith into which we've been welcomed. Readers will best appreciate the words (or concepts) and themes of this book if they have a foundation in the basic tenets of Catholic teaching. The Catholic Church was built on Truth Himself—Jesus Christ. Therefore, readers will grasp the significance of the topics most readily with a prior comprehension of what the Church imparts to us through Her infallible wisdom. Sacred Scripture, the *Catechism of the Catholic Church*, the Church's dogmatic teaching about the dignity of every human life, Her rich Tradition of virtue, and our own experiences form the underpinnings for the rationale, logical associations, and holy connections we make between God, our food, and all of life.

Foreword

In this book, Paula and Jennifer present a case. They seek to connect the whole-food plant-based (WFPB) diet movement with the Catholic faith. Like many others, they argue that a WFPB diet is better for human health, the poor, the unborn, animals, and the environment than our present standard American diet (SAD) or Western diet. The SAD—on which many of us were raised and to which we are so accustomed—is characterized by high amounts of meat, eggs, dairy, and processed food, as well as low consumption of whole foods, including fruits, vegetables, legumes, nuts, seeds, and whole grains. Leaving these whole foods out of the typical Western diet is unfortunate, as these are the healthiest foods on the planet for us, the foods that we have been designed to eat.

Over a year before I met Paula and Jennifer, I became convinced that taking on a WFPB diet was the healthiest and most virtuous, ethical, sustainable, and socially responsible way to eat. Although those making the WFPB diet case were never making the case from an explicitly Catholic perspective (the case was made on scientific and sometimes ethical grounds), I found many resonances with the teachings and ideals of the Catholic faith. For this reason, I took on this diet in early 2016. It also connected well with the original way of life of my religious order (the Order of Preachers, popularly known as the Dominicans), which involved not eating meat as a norm. I have never been healthier, and I have never felt better.

I have tried to share with others what I have found. In my pastoral counseling practice, I encourage a healthy lifestyle as a part of virtue and a life of holiness. To this end, I encourage people to eat a more plant-based diet. I also organized a film-discussion series in the summer of 2017 here at Saint Dominic Church in Washington, DC, called Faith & Food. It made a big impression upon the participants. Before the series began, Paula and Jennifer saw the series advertised and contacted me. We met and instantly found that we were simpatico on these matters. Our independent journeys resonated with each other, as did our enthusiasm to share what we discovered and what had so enriched us. All three of us had the desire to articulate the connections we saw and to attract Catholics and non-Catholics alike to a healthier and more virtuous and socially responsible way of eating. Paula and Jennifer graciously agreed to share their testimonies on the first night of the series. People loved and greatly benefited from their stories.

Of course, it isn't just the three of us who are undertaking this lifestyle change! More and more Catholics (as well as many people from other religious backgrounds) are discovering the benefits of a WFPB diet these days—or at least of a more plant-based diet, especially through the many works that Paula and Jennifer cite here, as well as through the popular documentary *Forks over Knives*. Many naturally see numerous connections to their faith and moral ideals. Paula and Jennifer have decided to take the extra step of articulating these connections in a published book. This might be a first.

It's an important step in helping Catholics look at and approach food differently.

Most people seem to make food choices on the basis of three things: (1) what tastes good to them, (2) what fills them up, and (3) what they are used to in their culture and personal habits. When what is healthy and sustainable tastes good, fills people, and is normative in cultural expectations and personal habits, these criteria are not a problem. The problem today is that what tastes good to people, what they think fills them up, and what they are used to in the Western culture is often unhealthy and promotes disease. In addition, the Western diet is unsustainable, and it has many negative effects on society, individuals, the health-care system, food laborers, families, the unborn, future generations, animals, and the environment. Most people are unaware of this ugly underbelly of our current conventional food system and culture. Most are also unaware of the many benefits that come with adhering to a better diet.

We Catholics are called to approach things from what is morally best—that is, what is God's will and what gives Him the greatest glory; what is best for the temple of the Holy Spirit that grace has made our bodies to become (1 Cor. 6:19–20); and what is best for our families, our society, the unborn, future generations, animals, and the environment. This is a very different approach to food than the one that those who adhere to the standard American diet undertake. It is approaching food through the lens of virtue, conscience, and Catholic social teaching.

We Catholics are called to choose conscience over convenience, long-term goods over fleeting pleasures, deeper goods over more shallow ones, and what is in accordance with the common good versus what is selfish. This is not an easy undertaking. We often put taste and convenience ahead of everything else. But Jesus calls us higher, even as He understands and helps us in our weaknesses through His mercy. When we let Him lead us, we can slowly overcome our addictions to unhealthy things. We can let Him help and strengthen us to choose what is best.

Paradoxically, we can actually enjoy food more than ever before. Indeed, one of the benefits of a WFPB diet is not only the satisfaction of conscience; it is also the satisfaction of enjoying some really delicious food (with a little experimentation with what works for you). Pleasure is not an end in itself. It shouldn't be sought for its own sake, apart from the deeper and more important good to which it is attached. Pleasure should be ordered to what is truly good. Yet pleasure is something that is naturally and fittingly attached to true goods. This is good news for us. Eating healthy and virtuously doesn't need to be—in fact, it *shouldn't* be—miserable. There is an abundance of delicious flavors in the plant kingdom. We certainly shouldn't become obsessive about food. Food is a means to so many other and more important aspects of life. When *what* we eat is good (a healthy, plant-rich diet), *why* we eat it is good (for God's glory and the good of others and ourselves), and *how* we eat it is good (gratefully, joyfully, hospitably, virtuously, and as a means toward growing in holiness), then we experience many levels of satisfaction that will fulfill us much more than any self-centered, momentary pleasure.

I invite you to prayerfully consider, with an open mind and heart, the case that Paula and Jennifer make here. Above all, ask Jesus—through the intercession of Mary and the saints—for the grace that you need to embrace and live out God's fulfilling will in all aspects of your life…including the area of food.

—Fr. Hyacinth Marie Cordell, OP
Parochial Vicar of St. Dominic Church in Washington, DC
September 20, 2017

Open Letter to Pope Francis

His Holiness, Pope Francis
Domus Sanctae Marthae
00120 Vatican City State

Dear Holy Father,

We are writing to you out of our deep love and compassion for our brothers and sisters around the world and for all of God's creation. We are troubled, as we know you are, about the millions of poor people who go hungry every day, about deteriorating human health, about skyrocketing medical costs, about environmental degradation, and about the culture of death. We have learned that eating animal-based foods is a fundamental cause of these concerns.

> And whoever gives only a cup of cold water to one of these little ones because he is a disciple—amen, I say to you, he will surely not lose his reward.
> —Matt. 10:42

The poor and hungry are particularly vulnerable to the (often unintended) consequences of our animal-based food system and to human corruption of food distribution systems. It may be surprising to learn that there is more than enough food to feed every person on the planet. We can feed the world simply by giving to humans the plenteous grains, vegetables, and fruits that are grown, instead of feeding them to animals raised for food. Animals eat much more food than they produce. They require food, water (2,500 to 4,000 gallons to produce a single pound of beef), medical care, and shelter...all at the expense of hungry people.

> Please test your servants for ten days. Let us be given vegetables to eat and water to drink. Then see how we look in comparison with the other young men who eat from the royal table...after ten days they looked healthier and better fed than any of the young men who ate from the royal table.
> —Dan. 1:12–15

The scientific evidence is overwhelming that consuming animals and their by-products is a key contributor to many of the world's chronic illnesses, such as heart disease, diabetes, obesity, high blood pressure, cancer, fibromyalgia, and beyond. A diet rich in animal-based foods is also implicated in human fertility and reproductive issues. And according to some studies, food is linked to early childhood diagnoses, such as attention deficit hyperactivity disorder (ADHD), attention deficit disorder (ADD), and autism.

The indigenous whole, starch-based foods (beans, potatoes, corn, rice, and other grains) that fed most humans for thousands of years are some of the healthiest foods on Earth. They have enabled civilizations to survive throughout the ages. Unfortunately, most of the planet has now adopted the rich Standard America Diet (SAD) of meat, dairy, eggs, refined grains, and junk food, resulting in a worldwide epidemic of chronic illness and obesity. Countless doctors, organizations, and scientists agree that diets rich in plant foods diminish disease and provide better nutrition than animal-based foods. Yet most people have never heard this well-documented information.

> In the beginning, when God created the heavens and the earth…God saw that it was good.
> —Gen. 1:1–25

The United Nations Food and Agricultural Organization reports that more global warming is caused by the meat industry than by all transportation combined (including cars, planes, trains, and other forms of transportation). In addition, the Worldwatch Institute states that animals raised for food account for *more than half* of all human-caused greenhouse gases. Furthermore, the Amazon rainforests are being destroyed to raise cattle for beef. We do not yet understand the long-term impacts of our decisions on the environment. We do know that eating a wholefood, starch- and plant-based diet is one of the most effective actions that we can take to reduce our environmental impact.

> Happy are you who sow before every stream, and let the ox and the donkey go freely!
> —Isa. 32:20

Factory farming is a cruel and incomprehensible system that we have thrust on the animals. The Catholic commentary in the New American Bible (NAB) regarding Genesis 1:29–30 states the following: "According to the Priestly tradition, the human race was originally intended to live on plants and fruits as were the animals, an arrangement that God will later change in view of the human inclination to violence." The Church doesn't excuse unnecessary violent behavior in any other area. Can She remain silent in this?

> God also said: See, I give you every seed-bearing plant on all the earth and every tree that has seed-bearing fruit on it to be your food.
> —Gen. 1:29

God, in His infinite wisdom and generosity, has given us all that we need for our nourishment and pleasure, but we have lost our way. Countless experts now believe that our world's health-care disaster, hunger crisis, and environmental devastation can begin to be reversed by changing our food choices. John McDougall, MD, best-selling author and nutrition expert, encouragingly says in *The Starch Solution*, "As luck would have it, the very same actions that can save your health and that of your loved ones will also mitigate the monumental environmental and food access problems that plague the world we live in." When God provides the solution, everyone can win.

As this information becomes more widely known, it is critical that people come together to address the issues related to the harmful animal-based food system. We believe that this is one of the most important pro-life issues affecting every stage of human life—from natural conception to natural death. We do not believe that the Church can remain passive at this point in history. While we recognize that these ideas represent a major societal shift, we believe that the Church can play a very important role in leading the flock to a deeper appreciation for creation and a greater awareness about how our food choices impact all stages and all forms of life.

> We know that all creation is groaning in labor pains even until now.
> —Rom. 8:22

We encourage you to consider this matter with the utmost care and discernment. We know that you have many challenges and issues to address, but this is an urgent matter because it affects all of life. What you have written in *Laudato Si* has done so much good, but much more needs to be done in this area. Perhaps you would consider assembling a working group to study these issues and to determine how to apply what is learned about food to the Church's life of virtue. We would be delighted to participate.

Most respectfully,

The Catholic Vegan Sisters

Paula B. Sandin Catholic Converts Vegan Converts	Jennifer S. Adams

INTRODUCTION

I have much more to tell you, but you cannot bear it now.
—John 16:12

Change the Food, Change the World. We have chosen to write about one of the most controversial and scorching hot-button issues of the human experience—diet. We learned that by changing the food we choose to eat, much of what ails the world can be healed, and—surprisingly—that *diet is directly linked to fostering a culture of life*. But not just any diet—a whole food, plant-based (WFPB) diet. So what *is* a WFPB diet? It simply consists of whole, plant foods, such as potatoes, beans, corn, rice (and other whole grains), fruits, and vegetables. We realize that our claim—that diet is so closely associated with life issues—probably sounds a bit strange, maybe even a little radical. However, in the following pages, we make the important, exciting, and holy connection between God, our food, and life.

We want to help promote and defend a culture of life. As Catholics, in order to be able to make wise decisions about anything, we know that it is important and necessary to have a well-formed conscience (based on faith and reason) "in conformity with the truth and good willed by the wisdom of the Creator" (according to #1783 in the *Catechism of the Catholic Church*). We must continually align our ways to His ways (based on principles found in the Bible and in the Catechism, and grounded in science) in order to more fully manifest a culture that protects, nourishes, and fosters human life. Human life is the pinnacle of God's creation because we are made in His image and likeness (Gen. 1:26). Yet a full expression of a culture of life encompasses *all* of creation—humans, the environment, and animals—because what God created is good (Gen. 1:31).

Sadly, much of the world is steeped in a culture of death. Disease, poverty, and destruction of human life (in all its stages) are considered normal. We are proposing that the proliferation of this culture of death is due, in many ways, to the foods that we eat. We want to change that. We believe that—with God's help—we have found a way to foster a culture of life through a WFPB diet. Until we change the food, the culture of life that we all desire will, in many aspects, remain elusive.

Through our life experiences and research (faith and reason), we discovered that our food choices touch every aspect of our society—whether we realize it or not—in obvious and subtle ways. The societal implications are rather staggering and easily recognizable once we identify the threads. Some of them are so obvious that we could hardly believe that we missed them for most of our lives. Science confirms that the food we eat is intricately and powerfully connected to the fruitfulness of humanity (human health, reproduction, our obligation to help the poor and hungry), the life of the planet (natural resources, weather patterns, ecosystems, rainforests), and the flourishing of the rest of God's creation (animals, crops, and all other living things). All parts of life are interconnected to one another and to the food that we eat. In fact, the food that we eat directly impacts, for good or bad, every aspect of life.

The foods that we have become most accustomed to eating in the last one hundred years (animal-based foods and processed foods) are more deleterious to our health and to our survival on Earth as a human race than many of us have recognized—*at least until now*. Starches and other plant-based foods comprised the traditional diets of all large healthy populations around the world for millennia.[1] Only recently (since the twentieth century) have we largely pushed those foods to the side (or slathered them with fats) and replaced them with ever-increasing quantities of meat, dairy, fish, eggs, and processed junk foods. These seemingly innocuous changes in the human diet of consuming vast amounts of animal proteins and fats have impacted society medically, socially, economically, morally, psychologically, environmentally, militarily, politically, and even religiously. Sadly, that impact includes chronic illness and obesity; overconsumption and misuse of natural resources; abuse of animals; a weakened military; and depriving the poor of the basic necessities of life, namely food and clean water. Yet starches and other plant-based foods remain the timeless answer for human health, environmental sustainability, and world hunger. The Bible begins (Gen. 1:29), continues (Ezek. 47:12), and ends (Rev. 22:2) the same way—with people eating plant-based diets for nourishment and healing, pointing to the foods that God provided for us out of His great love. Our society would change dramatically in countless ways if humans adopted a diet more in line with these scripture passages.

Our book is an attempt to illuminate the interconnectedness of making wise food choices to fostering a culture of life. We hope to unveil for you the reasons that returning to a traditional starch- and plant-based diet is one of the most significant answers to the positive changes that we seek in the world—and the one change that will more wholly foster the culture of life that God planned for us, the one that we all desire. While this is not your typical pro-life book, we have taken many of the Church's teachings on human life and demonstrated how we can uphold and support pro-life teachings most effectively by our food choices, often in surprising ways. We share the information that we have learned so that people can make well-informed decisions for themselves.

In the upcoming chapters, we identify key life concerns that are affected by our food choices: human health, reproduction and hormones, the poor and the hungry, the environment, and animals. While we do not have space in this book to explain the issues in extensive detail, we have tried to provide enough information to bring awareness and understanding so that our readers can pursue a more in-depth look at the issues. Because you are reading this book (by Divine appointment, of course), we believe that you will be interested in the holy connection that we make between God, our food, and life. Stay with us to discover how our food choices impact life in all of its forms.

Part I
Life Seeds

CHAPTER 1

Human Health

Life Seed: **Good health is critical for the flourishing of human life. However, human health is affected by poor food choices and can lead to chronic illness. This can prevent us from living fully and from using our God-given gifts and talents. It may also bankrupt us, steal our freedom, and prematurely end our lives.**

> Do you not know that your body is a temple of the Holy Spirit within you, whom you have from God, and that you are not your own?
> —1 Cor. 6:19

Human health compromised by chronic illness touches almost every person in some way, either directly or indirectly. If we aren't suffering from chronic illness ourselves, then we surely know someone who is. Chronic illnesses are those that are prolonged and are often assumed to have no cure. Some common chronic illnesses include obesity, heart disease, diabetes, high blood pressure, stroke, cancer, Alzheimer's disease, osteoporosis, and inflammatory arthritis.

The United States is experiencing an epidemic of these chronic diseases:

Obesity: 78.6 million people[2]
Heart disease: 27.6 million people[3]
Diabetes: 30.3 million people[4]
High blood pressure: 70 million people[5]
Stroke: 795,000 every year[6]
Cancer: >14 million people[7]
Alzheimer's: 5.4 million people[8]
Osteoporosis: 10 million people[9]
Inflammatory arthritis: 21 million people[10]

These illnesses are typically just "managed" by prescription pills, procedures, and potions, often with side effects as harmful as the illnesses themselves. We are told that this is the best that we can expect. Most of us don't know what else to do. Therefore, we accept and "live" with these illnesses, to lesser or greater degrees, for the rest of our lives. A great deal of suffering in our world is caused by these illnesses and is unwittingly self-inflicted. It may be surprising to learn that many chronic diseases are caused by poor lifestyle habits and that most of them are largely preventable.

Dietary Diseases (Our Modern-Day Plague)

> The doctor of the future will give no medication, but will interest his patients in the care of the human frame, diet and in the cause and prevention of disease.
> —Thomas Edison, American inventor and businessman

For the most part, chronic illnesses are dietary diseases. Wrong food choices, particularly animal-based and processed foods, are at the root of these illnesses. These foods are harming us. It may be shocking to learn that we're administering the poison ourselves each time we open our mouths to eat these foods. Chronic, degenerative disease is the result.

Examples of Chronic, Degenerative Diseases

Atherosclerosis: Clogged and damaged arteries from high cholesterol, high fat animal-based diets.
High blood pressure: The body's natural response to clogged and narrowing arteries as it works harder and harder to get the blood to and from the heart.
Cancer: Cell mutation, which can be *initiated* in numerous ways, including nutritional imbalances. Diet plays a chief role in cancer *promotion* and *progression*.[11]
Inflammatory arthritis: Inflammatory and degenerative condition linked to gut permeability ("leaky gut") caused by the acidic standard American diet (SAD).[12]

Diabetes: Insulin receptors clogged with fat, preventing insulin from getting into the cells resulting in insulin resistance.[13]
Alzheimer's disease: Clogged cerebral arteries from high fat diets (similar to heart disease), cutting off blood flow to the brain and leading to the development of Alzheimer's disease.[14]
Osteoporosis: Acidic condition in the body caused by animal-based diet. The body pulls calcium (a neutralizing agent) from the bones in order to neutralize the acid.[15]

Many believe that our genes are responsible for whether we contract these diseases, but that is an oversimplification. Genes can indicate a predisposition to disease, but they are *not always the final authority*. According to Dr. T. Colin Campbell, author of the famed book *The China Study*, genes are the foundation for everything that happens in the body, but it is the *food* that determines how those genes are expressed.[16] What an empowering and encouraging truth!

Human Food

> Their fruit is used for food, and their leaves for healing.
> —Ezek. 47:12

Many people don't realize that the right food choices can help us to prevent, even reverse, chronic diseases. **A whole food, starch- and plant-based diet is recommended by many of the leading medical doctors in the United States and around** the world today as the antidote to these illnesses.** Dr. John McDougall; Dr. Caldwell Esselstyn, Jr.; Dr. Neal Barnard; Dr. Thomas Campbell; Dr. Anthony Lim; Dr. Michael Greger; Dr. Kim Williams; Dr. Michael Klaper; Dr. Joel Fuhrman; Dr. Dean Ornish; Dr. Joel Kahn; Dr. Garth Davis; and hundreds of other doctors and nutrition experts advise people to avoid animal-based foods and unhealthy processed foods. Instead, they advocate a diet of whole plant-based foods for the prevention and reversal of many chronic diseases. We believe that we were divinely led to the truth about the power of eating a WFPB diet and that this truth needs to be shared so that others can benefit as we have. We, ourselves, experienced a total reversal of our chronic illnesses by adopting this way of eating (as chronicled in our book *Pick Up Your Mat…and Follow God to Divine Health through a Whole Food, Plant-Based Diet*).

Maybe this is the first time you've heard this information, and it seems foreign to you. We understand—we've been there. There are so many voices in our world today telling us what to eat, many of which are conflicting. Some "experts" say to eat high-protein diets for good health. Others say to consume "healthy" oils, and still others recommend eating fish to be healthy. Some experts recommend that we eliminate saturated fats from our diets (found primarily in animal-based foods), but we are then told, often by the same sources, that we need to consume animal protein (which contains high amounts of saturated fats). We are encouraged to eat more fiber, but then we hear that the very foods that contain fiber (like starches) will make us fat. There are many political and economic reasons that we receive these opposing recommendations, which we address later in the book. It can be very confusing until we go back to basics.

History

History and common sense can teach us a lot. Traditional diets of beans, potatoes, corn, rice (and other grains), fruits, and vegetables sustained large populations for many thousands of years.[17] Animal foods were seldom eaten, and if they were, they were only consumed in small portions. As a result, dietary diseases were rarely seen in populations of people who ate these traditional diets. There are still places on Earth where, by and large, people don't suffer from these illnesses. (For more information, read *The Blue Zones* by Dan Buettner.) However, those areas of the world are rapidly disappearing as more people gain access to the rich Western diet. For instance, Japanese and Chinese populations began to experience high rates of chronic illness only after adopting the standard American diet.[18] Asia imported processed products, fast food chains, and a penchant for animal foods to the detriment of its people. Chronic illnesses like heart disease, diabetes, cancer, high blood pressure, Alzheimer's disease, and osteoporosis were almost nonexistent in these populations, particularly in rural regions. In addition, chronic illnesses are largely modern phenomena caused by diets high in protein and fat from animal foods, oils (including so-called "heart-healthy" olive oil), and processed foods.[19] According to Rosane Oliveira, a researcher from the University of California, Davis, Department of Integrative Medicine, the Chinese people rarely suffered from diabetes until this increased consumption of animal-based foods. China now has diabetes rates similar to the United States.[20]

We read several historical accounts that fascinated us. During the Korean and Vietnam wars, autopsies conducted on young fallen US soldiers revealed a high rate of coronary heart disease. It is likely that autopsies of today's fallen soldiers would reveal the same (and probably worse) heart disease rates. Interestingly, also, during World War II, when European countries were occupied by the enemy, their cattle were confiscated. Innocent people were left with only legumes, potatoes, and other root vegetables to eat. On the surface, this might seem tragic. However, during this time, heart disease rates plummeted. After the war, when the people resumed their animal-based diets, previous rates of heart disease returned.[21]

The Protein Legend

One of the most predominant misconceptions in the field of nutrition today is that animal protein is critical for human health and that the more of it we consume, the better. Because meat has practically become synonymous with protein, it is hard for people to believe that protein is also found in plants. Widely held notions about animal protein are tied to physical strength and health. In addition, emotions regarding food are tied to deeply held family, religious, and cultural traditions. As a result of these beliefs and practices, even though the science is overwhelming and the evidence is compelling, many people will ignore—or outright reject—the information and die as a result of the chronic disease that they acquired from eating these foods.

Animal protein, historically considered higher-quality protein and more efficient for growth than vegetable protein, was once thought to be ideal for human health. However, further research has revealed that animal-based foods provide much higher levels of protein than we actually need. Further, we learned from the eCornell Nutrition Studies program that animal protein is so efficient for growth that it accelerates cancer cell growth and increases free radicals. Vegetable protein, on the other hand, is used in the body less efficiently than animal protein. This is actually a good thing, however, because vegetable protein promotes appropriate growth for human life and does not promote unwanted growth, such as cancer.[22]

One of the arguments against eating a plant-based diet is the myth that vegetable protein is incomplete in amino acids and therefore insufficient for human health. This myth advocates food combining to "make up" for the supposed incomplete amino acids. The myth in its entirety has been scientifically debunked many times but continues to be perpetuated in error today.[23] To be clear, vegetables do indeed contain all of the essential amino acids; thus, combining them is unnecessary. It is now known that a varied whole-food, starch- and plant-based diet (that contains enough calories) poses no threat of protein deficiency.

The recommended daily allowance (RDA) for protein can be calculated by using the following formula: body weight (kilograms) x 0.8 = grams of protein recommended per day. And this is even higher than many experts and doctors recommend. According to Dr. John McDougall, best-selling author and nutrition expert, most people need only 20 to 30 grams of protein per day. Regardless of the exact number, the amount of protein we need is easily obtainable from eating a variety of starches and other plant foods. Unfortunately, most of us are consuming far more protein than is healthy because of the Standard American Diet.[24]

> There are two kinds of cardiologists: vegans and those who haven't read the data.
> —Dr. Kim Williams, past president of the American College of Cardiology

The *Journal of the American Medical Association* reported on a study that revealed that "high animal protein intake was positively associated with cardiovascular mortality and high plant protein intake was *inversely* associated with cardiovascular and all-cause mortality."[25] Interestingly (and encouragingly), there is also evidence that a plant-based diet can help slow the aging process. *The Journal of Nutrition* published a Harvard Medical School study of fifty-four thousand women revealing that higher intakes of plant foods resulted in slower aging. The women who were followed for thirty years were more likely to "live independently and be free of physical limitations" if their diets were rich in fruits, vegetables, and walnuts.[26]

In addition to animal protein, animal fats and other fats (including "healthy" fats like olive and coconut oils) are problematic. Fats clog the body and make the blood sticky and sludge-like.[27] And processed foods, often containing animal and vegetable fats, may promote cancer.[28] Processed foods also often include high amounts of sugar, which can cause dangerous spikes in blood sugar. In addition, all of these foods (animal protein, fats, and processed foods) are virtually free of fiber and many life-giving nutrients.

Conversely, starches (such as potatoes, beans, corn, and whole grains) and other plant foods contain ideal levels of protein, carbohydrates, fats, micronutrients, and fiber—and they don't cause disease. We learned that they are, in fact, the perfect foods for human health. They don't burden the organs or other parts of the body, and they provide perfect nutrition for growth and human thriving, despite popular modern-day beliefs to the contrary. Starches are the foods we all crave—comfort foods. They satisfy us and are highly nutritious.[29] We lived the nightmare of life with chronic disease and found the key (with God's help) to excellent health—a whole-food, plant-based, oil-free diet.

> There are virtually no nutrients in animal-based foods that are not better provided by plants.
> —T. Colin Campbell, PhD, author of *The China Study* and *Whole*

Something Smells a Little Fishy

Fish, while being touted as a health food, can also be problematic. Many varieties of fish are high in cholesterol.[30] Additionally, many fish are contaminated with varying types and degrees of toxins. Farm-raised fish can contain antibiotics. Even wild-caught fish have been found to contain heavy metals (such as mercury) and noteworthy traces of prescription medications due to toxic dumping in the ocean and other waterways. In fact, salmon in the Puget Sound were found to contain eighty-one different substances, including prescription and over-the-counter drugs, as well as personal hygiene products.[31]

Many people eat fish because they are told that fish contain the right kind of fat—omega-3 fatty acids—and some fish do contain these essential fatty acids. But plant foods also contain an omega-3, namely alpha-linoleic acid (ALA). While ALA is only one of three omega-3 fatty acids, the human body is able to transform the ALA from plant foods into appropriate amounts of the other two omega-3 fatty acids, EPA and docosahexaenoic acid (DHA).[32] The good news is that we don't need to eat potentially toxic fish to get our omega-3s. Some plant foods high in ALA are walnuts, flaxseeds, chia seeds, and algae.

Obesity

It may surprise you to learn that many obese people, though over-fed, are starving from a nutritional standpoint. They are consuming calories with little to no nutritive value. Animal-based and processed foods don't contain many of the vitamins, minerals, and antioxidants that are essential to human health. We learned that hunger is the signaling message that the body uses to tell us that it needs nutrition. In addition to lacking nutrition, animal-based foods and processed junk foods contain no gut-filling fiber. Foods filled with fiber, such as starches, help us to feel full. Lack of satiety encourages overeating. If we eat fiber-less, nutrient-poor calories, our bodies will continue to signal to us that we need to consume more food.

The dieting cycle that we're all familiar with is one of deprivation and thus is not sustainable. Typical dieting practices that restrict calories and carbohydrates will never lead to permanent weight loss. Instead, when we eat the foods we love (such as starches), we become full and feel satisfied. This breaks the frustrating and unproductive cycle of deprivation and bingeing. The reason that whole-plant foods like starches contribute to weight loss is because, pound per pound, they are lower in calories than animal-based and processed foods. Dr. Anthony Lim, from the True North Health Center, laid out a rough estimate of various foods and their calories per pound.

Calories per Pound[33]

Food	Calories per Pound
Non-starchy vegetables	100
Fruit	300
Starches/whole grains	500
Legumes	600
Meat	1,000-1,100

Processed carbs (cereal, pasta)	1,200-1,300
Dried fruit	1,400
Sugar	1,500
Cookies	2,000
Nuts	2,800
Oils	4,000

According to Dr. Lim and others, as long as we eat foods that are 600 calories per pound or lower, we will effortlessly lose weight. As long as we don't add animal-based foods (such as dairy) and other fats (including extracted vegetable fats) to those foods, we will be able to eat whenever we are hungry and until we are satiated. The body will return to its natural God-given size when it is provided with the correct fuel. For more information, read *The Pleasure Trap* by Dr. Doug Lisle. (For those who are *not* struggling to lose weight, eating more processed starches like cereal, bread, and pasta can be part of a healthy plant-based diet. Also, dried fruits and nuts can be eaten in small amounts, but be forewarned…too much can quickly put on weight, to which we both can attest!)

> The fat you eat is the fat you wear.
> —Dr. John McDougall, physician, nutrition expert and best-selling author

Not only are many foods lacking in nutrition and fiber, but they are actually addictive. We learned from John and Ocean Robbins's *Food Revolution Summit* that the processed-foods industry intends for people to become addicted to their foods by incorporating addictive ingredients in their products. They even hire "crave-ability experts" to get consumers to crave their food products, and they do it by adding salt, oil, and sugar (SOS) to everything. The combination of these three ingredients is not found naturally in whole foods.[34] According to Dr. Robert Lustig, Professor of Pediatrics in the Division of Endocrinology at University of California, San Francisco, we don't have the capability to metabolize the amount of sugar in these foods, even though we love them and keep eating them.[35] Furthermore, these foods are convenient for us to obtain, and they often appear to be less expensive. However, this is only an illusion as they generally more expensive.

Mental Health

While we don't delve into the subject of mental health deeply in this book, we think that it's important to mention that when we eat the wrong foods, we may not feel as good mentally as we could or should. Think of how you might have felt right after lunch (during the afternoon slump) or after a big holiday meal. How we eat affects our brain in a wide range of ways and can cause illnesses from mild fatigue to depression. If you're anything like us, we didn't even know how badly we were feeling until we found out what it felt like to actually feel good. We had lived for so long with fatigue, brain fog, and the inability to concentrate that we thought that it was normal. We both consumed immense amounts of coffee just to drag ourselves through our daily activities.

We learned that starches and other plant foods provide perfect nutrition for the brain. According to Dr. McDougall, eating starches encourages higher serotonin levels in the brain, which results in less hyperactivity, depression, and anxiety.[36] The results of a study published in *PubMed* linked an increase in the consumption of fruits and vegetables to substantially greater happiness.

The research from universities in England and Australia showed that "increased fruit and vegetable consumption was predictive of increased happiness, life satisfaction, and well-being."[37] And some research has even shown that a WFPB diet can improve symptoms for those who have been diagnosed with ADHD and ADD, as well as those on the autism spectrum.[38] We are excited that we have witnessed the power of this in people we know, and we look forward to further research being done in this area. For optimal mental health, a plant-based diet seems to be best.

Health-Care Crisis

> People are fed by the food industry, which pays no attention to health, and are treated by the health industry, which pays no attention to food.
> —Wendell Berry, novelist, poet, and environmental activist

The United States is experiencing a severe health-care crisis, primarily because of dietary diseases. According to the CDC, more than 85 percent of all health-care costs are for people with one or more chronic illnesses.[39] Like most people, you probably have a family member, a friend, or a co-worker who suffers from one or more chronic diseases (or who has died from one). Perhaps you have a chronic dietary illness and you have experienced the financial hardships that accompany it. Health-care costs are bankrupting individuals, families, and nations. The United States' national health expenditure is more than three trillion dollars per year and costs an average of almost ten thousand dollars per year per person.[40] The United States has the highest per-capita expenditure on health care but ranks last among developed nations for health-care outcomes when it comes to chronic disease.[41] (It is worth noting, however, that the United States is among the most advanced when it comes to acute care—for example, treating broken bones and infectious diseases.)

Chronic illnesses are not the only diseases driving up health-care costs. According to the Physicians Committee for Responsible Medicine (PCRM) website, "Foodborne diseases cause an estimated 76 million illnesses, 325,000 hospitalizations, and 5,000 deaths in the United States each year."[42] Food-borne illnesses like salmonella, some strains of Escherichia coli (E. coli), and listeria are often transmitted by animals and their feces.[43] Food-borne illnesses, like those listed above, are not typically considered chronic diseases; they are acute diseases. Given that many of our chronic diseases are caused by the food that we eat, chronic diseases *are* themselves food-borne diseases. While they are not transmitted in the same ways as the previously mentioned food-borne diseases, they are no less dangerous, and they should be taken no less seriously.

> Heart disease is a food-borne illness.
> —Dr. Caldwell Esselstyn, physician and author of *Prevent and Reverse Heart Disease*

Despite all of the cutting-edge research, expenditure, medications, procedures, equipment, and popular lifestyle modifications typically recommended, chronic diseases increasingly plague us. Until we get the food right, these diseases will remain a part of our lives. The best science is on our side, and as mentioned previously, many doctors now recommend the WFPB diet. In fact, Kaiser Permanente, one of the nation's largest health-care providers, now encourages its network of doctors to recommend this way of eating to all of its patients.[44]

It's the food.
—Dr. John McDougall, physician, nutrition expert, and best-selling author

A Culture of Life or Death?
Chronic illnesses are not natural; they stem from the rich man's diet and have increased exponentially over the last hundred years as more people have access to and can afford animal-based and processed foods. Chronic diseases are stealing lives, bankrupting people and nations, and devastating families. We want to help people to avoid these illnesses—and the resulting consequences—and to understand that this is a human life issue that affects all of us is in many serious ways. Our acceptance of chronic illnesses as a normal state of human health and aging is one more way that society has bought into the prevailing culture of death.

Bishop Robert Barron offered an analogy of golf as it relates to the moral life. For anyone who plays golf, he explained, developing a correct golf swing can be a challenge because the wrong golf swing can *feel* so right, even if it's totally wrong. A golfer will continue to use an incorrect golf swing, even while it produces consistently bad results, simply because it feels right. He explained that the moral life is similar. Something may feel or seem right, even if it's morally wrong and will always produce negative results.

The same analogy that Bishop Barron used to explain the moral life can be used for our widely accepted animal-based, rich Western diet. We've been told all of our lives that we need to eat meat, dairy, fish, and eggs, and that these foods are healthy for us. We grew up on these foods. Our traditions were built around these foods. They *seem* right. Yet eating these foods consistently produces bad results, namely chronic diseases. Correcting a golf swing feels really awkward at first; however, after practicing with it for a while, it begins to feel comfortable, and sticking with it produces good results. The same could be said for switching to a whole-food, starch- and plant-based diet. It might seem different or strange in the beginning. However, once you begin to eat starches and realize how satisfying they are, how much better you feel, and how much more energy you have, adapting to it is very easy and can happen quickly. Taste buds adjust rapidly. And the icing on the cake (a healthy, plant-based one, of course!) is that the symptoms of chronic diseases can quickly begin to disappear with the adoption of a WFPB diet.

We want to help people to become well God's way and to fulfill their divine purpose on this earth. The *CCC* (#2288) says that we are to "take reasonable care" of ourselves because life and physical health are "precious gifts entrusted to us by God." It's important to note that eating whatever we want, regardless of the toll that doing so takes on our bodies, is *not* taking reasonable care of ourselves. On the other hand, adopting the whole-food, starch- and plant-based, oil-free diet is a key way to take reasonable care of ourselves. It is simple, it can be very inexpensive, and it provides the essential nutrients required for optimal human health. Chronic illnesses can be all-consuming, but when we adopt this healthier way of eating, we become well. We are then able to take the focus off of ourselves, our pains, our medical appointments, our procedures, our medications, our medical bills, and our debilitation. We can begin to live life more fully again.

> Some people think a plant-based, whole foods diet is extreme. Half a million people a year will have their chests opened up and a vein taken from their leg and sewn onto their coronary artery. Some people would call that extreme.
> —Dr. Caldwell Esselstyn, physician and author of *Prevent and Reverse Heart Disease*

Eradicating or minimizing chronic disease is not an attempt to live forever or to unnaturally prolong life. After all, we *want* to be with the Lord in His glory forever. And we know that we must all experience death. As Catholics, we die with the hope that we will be raised with Christ and live with Him in eternity. The *Catechism* (#1014) even tells us that we can and should pray for a happy death. In fact, Saint Joseph is the patron of a happy death. Not only can we pray for a happy death, but we can eat in a way that increases our chances of experiencing a happy death. Contrast that with the agony and indignities of death caused by chronic illness. People with brilliant, sharp, and creative minds still full of the desire to live are hampered by disintegrating and failing bodies that are wracked with diseases. And physically active people who succumb to severe dementia and Alzheimer's disease continue to "live" in their able bodies without a sound mind. In all of these cases, the standard American diet is largely to blame. It is all so sad and unnecessary.

Another terrible side effect of our modern-day diets and resulting illnesses is that people want to relieve themselves of the dreadful physical suffering that they experience by any means possible. Some try to gain relief with prescription pills (such as opioids) or with medical marijuana, which can initiate a whole host of other problems. In extreme cases, people want to end their own lives. Of course, the Catholic Church is steadfastly opposed to any action that intentionally hastens or unnaturally ends life. Might the increasing trend and desire for doctor-assisted suicide (and other forms of euthanasia) decline if painful chronic diseases disappeared?

What more ingenious way for the devil to destroy humanity and the rest of God's beautiful creation than with food? Food is critical; we all need it, and we all desire and crave it. But our forks and knives have become weapons that we use to inflict harm on ourselves. The devil tempts us, and we take the bait…literally. Our enemy is hidden in plain sight.

> Homicide is 0.8% of deaths. Diet-related disease is over 60%. But no one talks about it.
> —Jamie Oliver, British celebrity chef

Suffering

> The devil has put a penalty on all things we enjoy in life. Either we suffer in health, or we suffer in soul, or we get fat.
> —Albert Einstein, physicist

Can we fulfill God's highest purpose for us if we're sick? Maybe, but if we're distracted by illness, pain, and debilitation, it will be difficult at best. According to Bishop Barron, sickness draws us into and around ourselves. Wellness allows us to serve and "to be for the other."[45] We can use our illness for good, to get closer to God, and to offer our redemptive suffering to God, but we have to ask ourselves if God might offer us another path. We don't believe that sickness is a "cross" *given* to us by God. Instead, we believe that God *allows* illness and suffering and can use it to bring about a greater purpose. Suffering is a part of human life, and we have been told to expect it. But illness is not the pinnacle of the life experience, and it is certainly not *from* God. (If that were the case, wouldn't seeking any medical attention be disobedient to God's will?)

While we acknowledge that suffering can be a gift (and that we can often benefit from and use it for our spiritual growth and for the good of others), we believe that some suffering is unnecessary. None of us would tell someone to continue to smoke cigarettes. We know that smoking can lead to emphysema, lung cancer, and heart attacks, along with a great deal of suffering. This could be considered unnecessary suffering because we have the ability to make the choice *not* to smoke. It works the same way with the food. Illness is often a result of our own poor or uninformed food and lifestyle choices. Our real cross may be to make difficult lifestyle changes, to do what it takes to become healthy, and then to be a witness of wellness and a changed life to the world. God, through the Church, has counseled us to a life of temperance, fortitude, simplicity, and fasting. The rich Western diet and the gluttony that it perpetuates fly directly in the face of that guidance.

The Church places a great deal of emphasis on human dignity. Unfortunately, people suffering from chronic illnesses often become defined in the medical system by their diseases and are not treated as whole persons, or with dignity. In addition, we often see people with chronic diseases define *themselves* in terms of their illness. Their whole lives are arranged around the illness, as we know only too well. Being entwined in the medical system can exacerbate fear, and we can forget that we don't need to panic. It's important for people to remember who they really are—they are not just a set of symptoms. We want to encourage people to live their lives and to have fun, even if they are dealing with a medical condition. We also want to encourage people—while they're living their lives—to seek God's guidance and to consider pursuing avenues of healing through proper nutrition. *Stay open,* as God counseled us.

The root of suffering is attachment.
—Buddha, ascetic and sage

Food for Thought:

1. *Prior to reading this chapter, did you know that many chronic diseases are caused by eating animal-based and processed foods? Were you surprised by anything that you learned?*
2. *Are you concerned about chronic disease? What changes would you have to make in your own diet to improve your health and to avoid chronic illness?*
3. *Do you know of anyone suffering with a chronic disease? Can you identify the types of foods that might be contributing to that person's illness? Would you feel comfortable sharing the information you've learned to help that person?*
4. *Are you glad that you have been given this information that can potentially help you and your loved ones to avoid or to heal from many chronic diseases? What about this information is encouraging to you? Do you have any concerns?*
5. *Now that you know that animal-based foods are not necessary for human health, do you consider a plant-based diet to be a valid option for you?*
6. *What specific steps might you be interested in taking toward learning more about the health benefits of a whole food, plant-based, oil-free diet? (Some examples include watching* Forks

over Knives, *reading* The Starch Solution, *and enrolling in the eCornell Plant-Based Nutrition course.)*
7. *If you are struggling with weight loss, does the calories-per-pound chart in this chapter give you any encouragement?*

CHAPTER 2

Reproduction and Hormones

Life Seed: Reproduction is essential for bringing about future human life. The health of mothers and fathers is closely tied to reproductive outcomes and can greatly affect life at all levels—individual, societal, and global—for good or for bad. Hormones, which are the body's messengers, are linked to reproduction, as well as to other vital functions of the body.

> You formed my inmost being; you knit me in my mother's womb. I praise you, because I am wonderfully made.
> —Ps. 139:13–14

The Catholic Church, in Her great wisdom and fullness, recognizes that life is the most precious gift that we have been given. After all, God created life—He is life itself. God's beautiful plans for life are found throughout the pages of the Bible and are illuminated in the *Catechism of the Catholic Church (CCC)*. Gen. (1:27) tells us that God created man and woman in His likeness and image. In His generosity, God has given human beings a share in the creation of life through the conjugal act of love in the bond of marriage. Gen. (2:24) and the *CCC* (#372) teach that, in marriage, God unites a man and a woman, and they become one flesh. After this holy union, man and woman are called to be fruitful and multiply, and to fill the earth (Gen. 1:28). In this, the *Catechism* says, we are cooperating in a unique way in the Creator's work.

Modern man has drifted from God and His blueprint for life, reproduction, and sexuality. While it is common for humans to doubt in God's perfect plan, the divine plan for reproduction and sexuality is a pretty simple (though sometimes challenging) one to follow. Ideally, reproduction results in healthy pregnancies and babies, but far too often, it doesn't. Might something be thwarting God's perfect plan? We discovered that eating the wrong foods—foods that don't promote health—may be culpable for many reproductive problems. We offer two possible causes for consideration: (1) Reproduction, sexuality, and related outcomes are dependent on hormones. Animal-based foods are laden with natural and added hormones. Animal hormones are different from human hormones, and they may interfere with reproduction and (2) Dead foods (such as decaying animal-based foods and processed foods) do not provide the proper nutrition for human bodies and therefore are not optimal for reproduction or its outcomes.

We recognize that reproduction and hormones are very much a part of human health and could have been covered in the first chapter. However, we chose to address them in a separate chapter to underscore the significance of each topic as they relate to pro-life principles. The following sections in this chapter include, but are not limited to, ways in which reproduction and hormones are affected by the foods that we eat.

Endometriosis

During a woman's monthly menstrual cycle, endometrial tissue builds up in the uterus and sheds, resulting in bleeding. Endometriosis occurs when some of this endometrial tissue grows outside of the uterus. It often causes pain, inflammation, heavy periods, and infertility.[46] A side effect of endometriosis is the growth of cysts on the ovaries.

Endometriosis is often caused by a high-fat diet of animal-based foods, particularly dairy, and can be largely cured by adopting a WFPB diet.[47] (You can read about Jennifer's painful experiences of endometriosis and ovarian cysts—and healing by a change in diet—in our book *Pick Up Your Mat...and Follow God to Divine Health through a Whole Food, Plant-Based Diet*.)

Erectile Dysfunction

Erectile dysfunction is often called the canary in the coal mine because it points to a more serious underlying condition, namely heart disease.[48] The human body is an arterial system (arteries run through all of our organs, including the penis and vagina). When arteries, such as those in our chest, are clogged with fat and cholesterol, blood flow is impeded, and we suffer from all manner of heart disease. The smaller vessels in our sex organs are affected first, even before the larger arteries. The blockage in these smaller vessels and the resulting lack of blood flow prevent the normal effects of erection and ejaculation. This life-saving information is not widely known by the general population. Men are often directed to prescription medications, instead of what can really help—a primarily plant-based diet.[49]

Infertility

Couples who discover that they are sterile suffer greatly. In the Bible, Sarai was childless because she was not able to conceive (Gen. 11:30). "Lord God, what can you give me, if I die childless?" asks Abraham (her husband) of God (Gen. 15:2). But with God's blessing, Sarah was able to conceive in her old age (Gen. 21:6). In addition, Rachel cried to her husband, Jacob, "Give me children, or I shall die!" (Gen 30:1) In marriage, not all couples have the blessing of achieving pregnancy. And many couples who do conceive do so with much difficulty (*CCC* #2374).

Infertility and difficulty conceiving can have numerous causes. One cause is the less-than-optimal health of the mother and/or father. Poor health affects the viability of the mother's eggs and the father's sperm. Sadly, many men and women are not healthy enough to procreate by natural means, if at all. These struggling couples, especially young couples, may not even know that they are unhealthy because neither has any overt symptoms. But poor nutrition from diets that are high in animal-based foods and low in plant-based foods impacts every part of the body, including the reproductive system. Obesity, endometriosis, erectile dysfunction, high estrogen levels, and low testosterone levels, among others, can greatly affect a couple's ability to reproduce and can all be caused by eating the wrong foods. "The rich Western diet changes female hormones and as a result causes the development of disease in tissues that are hormone dependent—those of the uterus, ovary, vagina, and breast," says Dr. McDougall.[50]

As a result, couples who are desperate to have children often turn to unnatural means, such as artificial insemination or in vitro fertilization (IVF). They don't understand—and have never been told—that they may not be healthy enough to reproduce and that a change in diet might make a difference before they have to consider more drastic means. In vitro fertilization works by implanting embryos in the mother's womb. Only certain eggs and sperm are used to create the embryos, requiring the disposal of the remainder of embryos. This practice is not recognized by the Church as a morally acceptable process or outcome (*CCC* #2377). Overall, success rates of IVF range only between 13 and 43 percent.[51] In any case, embryos (preborn human beings) are lost during this procedure.

The *Catechism* (#2375) states, "Research aimed at reducing human sterility is to be encouraged, on condition that it is placed at the service of the human person, of his inalienable rights, and his true and integral good according to the design and will of God." Trying to determine how different eating patterns affect pregnancy, infertility, and sterility would not only be a worthwhile research effort but, we believe, a crucial one. Some research has already been conducted in this area. According to Dr. Michael Greger, "Meat is so packed with sex steroid hormones that when pregnant women eat meat it may affect the development of their sons' genital organs while still in the womb such that when he grows up he may have decreased fertility."[52] In addition, it has been established that eating meat causes a dramatic drop in male testosterone within three hours of eating a high-fat meal of animal meats. Conversely, eating plant foods increases testosterone levels.[53]

The famed Harvard nurses' study of one hundred and sixteen thousand nurses revealed a detrimental link between animal protein intake and ovular infertility. One serving of meat per day was associated with a 30 percent increase in infertility, while an increase in vegetable protein was associated with a "substantially lower risk of ovulatory infertility."[54] According to Dr. McDougall, switching to a low-fat, plant-based diet can help a woman's reproductive system to correct and heal itself.[55]

Stress

Research reveals that pregnant women who eat more meat and fewer vegetables experience an increase in stress hormones, which affect their babies' stress hormones and can impact their children's ability to cope with stress even as they become adults.[56] As previously mentioned, plant foods reduce these stress hormone levels. They also reduce depression. According to the PCRM, depression is linked to low serotonin levels and inflammation in the body. Plant foods raise serotonin and reduce inflammation.[57]

Babies and Children

The healthiest food for human babies is human breast milk because it contains the nutrients and antibodies required for optimal nutrition and immunity. Human breast milk was made for human babies. Farm animal milk was made for farm animal babies, not human babies (or human adults, for that matter). Numerous well-known doctors who are experts in nutrition and human health support feeding a vegan diet to children once they are weaned. A vegan diet containing sufficient calories is the healthiest diet for children and adults alike.[58] The Academy of Nutrition and Dietetics agrees, citing the vegan diet as the healthiest for all stages of life, including pregnancy and infancy.[59]

Acne

Powerful teenage hormones, combined with hormones from animal-based foods, set the body up for acne. According to Dr. Michael Greger, "Dairy is considered a major cause of the acne epidemic…by widespread cow milk consumption."[60] He illuminates several studies that make a connection between acne and dairy consumption, which point to sex steroid hormones present in cows' milk as the culprit. Populations that don't consume dairy products don't have the acne problems that Western nations do.[61] Other foods of the standard American diet, including those that are heavy in oils and processed foods, also contribute to acne problems.[62]

We all know that acne affects the self-esteem of young people who want to appear attractive as they seek a suitable mate. Sadly, a disturbing treatment has been practiced for many years—doctors have prescribed birth control pills to teenage girls as an antidote for acne. Unfortunately, there are many possible damaging side effects of the pill for all women, including these young teens. Young male teens who also experience embarrassing acne are often treated with harsh steroids. Fortunately, we know from experience that these drastic measures are unnecessary. When Jennifer's son was a teenager, he eliminated his acne in just three days by ditching all dairy products and, as a result, became vegan. Many others have seen similar results.

Human Sexuality and Promiscuity

We learn from the CCC (#2332) that "sexuality affects all aspects of the human person in the unity of his body and soul." This sexuality is largely controlled by our hormones, which become especially prominent in the teenage years. Teenage promiscuity in our current culture is rampant, and sexual activity is becoming normal for even the youngest of teens. During the teenage years, hormones are raging. Our children have grown up eating and drinking immense amounts of meat and dairy products, all of which are saturated with animal hormones.

Dairy is produced from the milk of lactating female cows. New mothers, human or otherwise, produce milk needed to feed their babies so that they will grow. In the case of a dairy cow, once she delivers, her calf is taken from her so that her milk can be used for human consumption. (The calf, if male, is discarded for slaughter or put into a veal crate. If female, she is raised for mass reproduction for the purpose of taking her calf's milk.) The milk that we take from the dairy cow is filled with hormones intended to quickly grow her calf into a six hundred-pound cow. Those are just the *naturally* occurring hormones, not to mention any *added* hormones. Putting these hormones (natural or otherwise) into young human bodies encourages unnatural growth, physically and sexually. For example, menstruation is occurring several years earlier in girls than it was only a couple of decades ago.[63]

According to Dr. McDougall, "As populations of people have gradually changed their diets from plant-based to animal-based (rich in meats, dairy products, and refined foods), the onset of sexual maturity has decreased at a rate of about 2 to 6 months per decade."[64] The concern with this is that the earlier in life people mature sexually, the younger they may become active sexually. For many, this has led to unwanted pregnancies and abortions (not to mention the epidemic of sexually transmitted diseases). This may be one of a number of reasons for the increased use of contraceptives and abortifacients.

Same-Sex Attraction and Gender Identity

There is another sensitive issue that we would like to address regarding food. Might it be possible that food, at least in part, is affecting our sexual inclinations and identities? We are not scientists, but it seems perfectly plausible to us that eating animal-based foods full of hormones and chemicals could alter, damage, or confuse our own hormones and genes. After all, eating animal-based foods has been shown to alter and damage our body chemistry in other ways, especially in ways that lead to disease.

Is it also possible that what parents eat before conceiving and what mothers eat while pregnant could affect their child's sexuality? (As stated before, we know that a pregnant mother's diet can affect her unborn baby and its future health in significant ways.) Many people who grapple with issues of sexuality say that they have been born in those ways and would rather not have to struggle with same-sex attraction or gender identity challenges. Isn't it worth considering if food could be causing sexual problems for many people? We are not being judgmental. We are simply raising questions and seeking answers to these and other difficult matters. We believe that further discussion and research would be valuable.

Toxic Burden

According to Dr. McDougall, high levels of environmental chemicals are also among the biggest dangers to successful reproduction. Bioaccumulation in the food supply is the process whereby substances (chemicals, in this case) become more concentrated (toxic) the higher you go on the food chain. For example, chemicals are sprayed on plants. Then, animals eat the plants. Next, the chemicals are stored in concentrated amounts in the animals' muscles and fat. Finally, humans eat the animals, along with the stored chemicals.

Thus, upward of 90 percent of environmental chemicals are found in animal-based foods because animals (who consume these chemicals in their feed) are high on the food chain where chemical concentration is higher. These chemicals can damage human deoxyribonucleic acid (DNA), cause birth defects, and wreak havoc on hormones.[65] Therefore, it makes sense that humans eating low on the food chain (organic plant foods) can avoid more of these toxins.

Love + Plants = Life

Pro-lifers, if they were aware of the issues we cover in this chapter, might become the strongest advocates for a WFPB diet.

> The food you eat can be either the safest and most powerful form of medicine or the slowest form of poison.
> —Ann Wigmore

Food for Thought:

1. Had you ever thought about the fact that humans regularly consume the naturally produced hormones of other animals when they eat animal-based products? (Examples of these products include cheese, milk, yogurt, ice cream, and meat.)
2. In your opinion, should couples struggling with infertility be given information by their doctors about how adopting a plant-based diet might help them to conceive and have healthy babies?
3. If you were struggling with infertility, would you be willing to adopt a WFPB diet before pursuing more drastic means?
4. Were you surprised to learn that dairy consumption is associated with acne? Do you know of anyone who might benefit from this information?
5. Do you think it is plausible that human consumption of animals (and therefore their hormones) might be affecting human sexuality and other hormone-dependent functions?

CHAPTER 3

THE POOR AND THE HUNGRY

Life Seed: The poor and the hungry are in our midst near and far. Their lives are of the utmost importance to God. The Church holds the poor in the highest esteem and requires the faithful to humbly serve and love the poor in all ways to the best of our ability.

> For I was hungry and you gave me food, I was thirsty and you gave me drink.
> —Matt. 25:35

Most people around the world are poor—materially poor—compared with those in the United States. That's hard to imagine from an American perspective. Many people in the world don't have adequate housing, clothing, or education. But the worst of it is that many don't have enough food to eat or water to drink. And if they do have food, it's often unhealthy; if they have water, it is often contaminated. Unbelievably, one in eight people around the world are underfed.[66] This inexcusable crime (sin) against humanity goes on while US food consumption is at an all-time high, consisting of diets heavy in animal products, salt, oil, and sugar (SOS).

Americans, on average, eat more calories per day than ever before. Daily calorie consumption increased between 1970 and 2008 by approximately 23 percent.[67] Compare that to the rest of the world that often does not have enough to eat.

In response to the shortfalls, the United States sends food around the world. However, our well-intentioned attempts to help the poor and hungry by sending our rich Western diets to other countries have produced unintended consequences. We have essentially exported chronic disease to the poor and other vulnerable populations. In addition, they have adopted our dietary and farming practices, which have often resulted in over-farmed lands, increased water pollution, and the exploitation of natural resources. These are just a few of the inadvertent costs.

Understanding these unintended costs is critical to finding the best solutions to feed our hungry world responsibly and is directly linked to our care for the poor. Offering the proper nutrition of a WFPB diet would help to diminish disease and reduce cost. It would also allow for precious water and land to be used for growing plant-based foods for human consumption, rather than for food to feed to farm animals. In addition, plant-based farming would help to reduce unnecessary water contamination caused by animal-waste runoff.

Hunger and Malnutrition

Our current food system, including production and distribution, is falling short. The agricultural system and our appetite for animal-based foods are contributing to problems of hunger, starvation, and malnutrition around the world. Using land and water resources to raise animals (and to grow their feed), instead of using the same resources to grow organic plant foods for human consumption, is highly counterproductive to adequately feeding our nation and our world. As stated previously, animals eat much more food than they produce. And they require food, water (2,500 to 4,000 gallons to produce one pound of beef), medical care, and shelter... all at the expense of our hungry brothers and sisters.[68] According to the United Nations, a child dies of hunger somewhere in the world every five seconds.[69] This, we have come to understand, is primarily because of inefficiencies and corruption in distribution, as well as the Western appetite for animal foods. Further, the documentary *Cowspiracy* reports, "82 percent of starving children live in countries where food is fed to animals, and the animals are eaten by Western countries."[70]

Even in the United States, as hard as it is to believe, hunger and malnutrition are present in many communities. Healthy foods are not always readily available to the poorest in our country. For example, in many inner cities, grocery stores have abandoned countless neighborhoods due to economic shortages and crime. What is left in their place are fast food chains that tend to serve processed and animal-based foods, which are linked to chronic disease. People in these communities, while often consuming an excessive number of calories, tend to be obese—as well as malnourished—from a lack of nutritional food options, as mentioned previously. Furthermore, there are poor communities that don't even have access to fast food.[71] As a side note, we have both witnessed another very concerning trend. On several occasions, we have seen people use their Supplemental Nutrition Assistance Program (SNAP) cards in convenience stores to buy groceries. These food products tend to be expensive, processed, and unhealthy.

Fast food = fast death.
—The Fresh Quotes

Food and Water Shortages

> And whoever gives only a cup of cold water to one of these little ones to drink because he is a disciple—amen, I say to you, he will surely not lose his reward.
> —Matt. 10:42

Population control is cited by some as the answer to our food and land shortage problems around the world. However, the problem is not with human overpopulation but with farm animal overpopulation. Up to *80 percent of all agricultural land* (or 50 percent of all land) is used in some way to grow animals for food or to grow animal feed.[72] To improve our chances for having enough space in the world for our growing population, we have to make different choices about how, and for what purposes, we use our land.

John Robbins, in his landmark book *Diet for a New America*, reveals that animals grown for food consume an amount of food greater than the caloric needs of the entire human population of the planet.[73] We can begin to feed the world simply by giving to humans the plenteous grains, fruits, and vegetables that are grown, instead of feeding them to animals.

According to A Well-Fed World (AWFW), a worldwide, nonprofit organization targeting hunger relief and animal protection, it takes as much as ten times the amount of water to grow animals as it does to grow crops for human food.[74] In poor and drought-stricken nations, scarce water resources are often given to animals or to grow animal feed. *Cowspiracy* reports that "animal agriculture is responsible for twenty to thirty-three percent of all fresh water consumption in the world today."[75] Adopting the Western diet of animal foods requires these nations to be in direct competition for drinking water with the animals, according to AWFW. In these poor countries, animals drink out of (and defecate in) the same streams from which the people drink. Diseases spread quickly, and many people get sick or die as a result.

Another concern is that conventional crop farming practices may be restricting food access. Current conventional practices of irrigation, single-crop planting, and the use of pesticides result in soil degradation, erosion, and pollution, which we fear produces less food. Interestingly, according to the United States Conference of Catholic Bishops (USCCB), "[Indigenous] technologies are more compatible with the ecosystem, are more available to poor persons, and are more sustainable for the entire community."[76] Organic farming practices can enable higher crop yields while restoring depleted lands. And during drought conditions, organically grown corn produces 33 percent more than conventionally grown corn; organically grown soy produces 50 percent more.[77] The good news seems to be that the simpler the method, the greater and better the output.

Food Subsidies

Currently in the United States, animal-based food agriculture is heavily subsidized. What's more, the US government buys millions of dollars' worth of surplus dairy and eggs to artificially prop up the egg and dairy industries. The government then funnels these animal products into food banks and other food assistance programs, including public school lunches.[78]

We believe that we can use our resources much more efficiently to help feed a starving world. Perhaps subsidies for US organic plant-based farming would be better, instead (if any food subsidies are needed at all). As a result, the *real* prices of animal-based foods would rise dramatically, and people would naturally eat less of these foods. In response, people might turn to healthier foods. Organic plant foods would go down in price and would further encourage healthier eating. Fortunately, US consumer demand for animal-based products is already waning, while interest in vegan alternatives is increasing.[79] Consumer demand for organic fruits and vegetables is also increasing.

Our Moral Obligation

>   Love is feeding everybody.
>   —John Denver[80]

As Catholics, we know that we have a moral obligation to feed the poor and give drink to the thirsty, which are the first two corporal works of mercy. We also know that faith apart from works is dead (Jas. 2:17). And we learn from Sacred Scripture that all are members of the Lord's body. (1 Cor. 12:27). However, many in our world believe that the poor and hungry of the Earth are someone else's problem. It is easy to become complacent, particularly when many of us have never witnessed or experienced poverty or hunger ourselves. When the destitute are out of our sight, they can be easily forgotten—out of sight, out of mind. Even when we want to help, we might not know what to do.

American Catholics and other people of goodwill generously try to help by giving money to governments (through our taxes) and charitable organizations, which distribute tons of food annually to poverty-stricken areas. However, throwing money at the problem does not require action or change from us as individuals. Instead, we mostly depend on others to buy and distribute food and water to the poor. Despite these huge efforts and money invested, the problems are still not solved. Though we know from Jesus that we will always have the poor with us (Matt. 26:11), we know that we can do better! What, then, might we do to help?

As we stated before, grains that could be used to feed the hungry often go to feed animals. Food crops, such as grains, have a much greater food relief impact, provide better nutrition, and yield greater health outcomes than do animal-based foods. With this knowledge, are we willing to take the more challenging action of changing our diet and reducing (or completely giving up) our animal-based foods to help feed the hungry? In other words, as prudence teaches us, are we willing to sacrifice lower goods for higher goods, as the Catholic Church commends? (Thankfully, we can still enjoy our favorite delicacies by replacing them with foods and treats made with yummy plant-based ingredients.) This might require a seemingly difficult sacrifice but it would greatly benefit us, our planet, and our brothers and sisters around the world. Transitioning to a WFPB diet provides for more efficiency and better health, and it makes a real impact for the hungry and poor.

> ...vast swaths of the world population suffer from malnourishment and starvation while those of us living in prosperous western nations indulge in our favorite foods.
>
> —Dr. John McDougall, physician, nutrition expert, and best-selling author

Food for Thought:

1. *If you were assured that widespread adoption of a WFPB diet would help the poor and hungry around the world, would you be willing to try it? What sacrifices would you have to make in order to do so?*

2. In addition to what was mentioned in this chapter, how might the poor and hungry benefit from a worldwide transition to a plant-based diet? What creative ways of plant-based farming and eating could be developed to benefit poor people worldwide?
3. Have you ever given money to an animal-gifting charity? Can you see how giving animals to a poor community might become problematic for the community? Would you be interested in giving to an all plant-based food charity and/or a clean water charity?
4. As a taxpayer, do you believe that school lunches, especially in vulnerable populations, should include healthier food options for students? What benefits do you perceive there to be in doing so? What might be the challenges?

CHAPTER 4

THE ENVIRONMENT

Life Seed: **Human beings have been given responsibility for the Earth and all that lives within it. Life can work out best for us when our choices about creation and all living creatures are made respectfully, in cooperation with the guidance of the Holy Spirit, and in accord with God's divine law for the benefit of human life.**

> The human family is charged with preserving the beauty, diversity, and integrity of nature, as well as with fostering its productivity.
> —United States Conference of Catholic Bishops[81]

The Catholic Church has recognized that our planet is experiencing severe stress. We have a choice—as a worldwide community—about how, or whether, to address the growing environmental challenges facing humanity. Our most recent popes have shared their own thoughts about the issues.

Pope Saint John Paul II: "Faced with the widespread destruction of the environment, people everywhere are coming to understand that we cannot continue to use the goods of the earth as we have in the past."[82]

Pope Benedict XVI: "The Church has a responsibility towards creation and she must assert this responsibility in the public sphere. In so doing, she must defend not only earth, water and air as gifts of creation that belong to everyone. She must above all protect mankind from self-destruction."[83]

Pope Francis: "[The Earth] now cries out to us because of the harm we have inflicted on her by our irresponsible use and abuse of the goods with which God has endowed her."[84]

As Catholics, we are urged to consider and take seriously what our holy fathers and bishops have said. Whether or not we believe that human-induced climate change or global warming is real, most people can find value in the idea of taking better care of the Earth and using our natural resources more wisely. The Earth, its resources, and the many creatures that call it home have been given to us by God to enjoy and to use respectfully for our benefit. There is not a person on the planet who has not recognized some beauty in nature or been in awe of some aspect of God's handiwork. Think of a starry night, a frothy ocean, snow-capped mountain peaks, rushing waterfalls, or any other everyday marvel that fills up our senses with wonder and joy.

The Earth is for us and for our well-being. It is not an albatross or a burden. It is our home, and everyone wants to live in a nice home. God created it tailor-made for us humans and for all forms of life. It comprises the perfect air for our lungs, the perfect water for our thirst, and the perfect food for our health and enjoyment. The sun is the perfect distance from the Earth for our light and our warmth. And the other creatures of the Earth are things of wonder and beauty with their own purposes and with whom we get to share the planet to our mutual advantage. What a gift we have all been given.

__Stewardship__

> God looked at everything He had made, and found it very good.
> —Gen. 1:31

God gave us dominion over the Earth (Gen. 1:26), and the way in which we define the word "dominion" will determine how we ultimately treat our planet. We believe that dominion implies stewardship and that we were given great responsibility for God's creation. If we can step aside from the political issues related to the environment, it seems to us that almost everyone would agree that it is completely to our benefit as humans to treat Earth and all of its inhabitants with goodness and gentleness. Unfortunately, our modern standard American diet and current food system are at odds with good stewardship in several ways.

__Animal Agriculture__

Although many people may not know this, modern animal agriculture is one of the leading causes of environmental destruction. According to the United Nations, more global warming is caused by the meat industry than by all transportation combined (including cars, planes, trains, and other forms of transportation).[85] And according to the Worldwatch Institute, animals raised for food account for *more than half* of all human-caused greenhouse gases.[86] It may be surprising to learn that an enormous amount of methane gas is produced in the animal agriculture sector and that cow flatulence accounts for one hundred and fifty billion gallons of methane gas produced per day worldwide.[87] Why does this matter? God fashioned a finely tuned atmosphere for life on Earth. Do we really know how much latitude we have in atmospheric fluctuations before our planet is out of balance and becomes incompatible for our survival? We don't know the answer, but we believe that God created the perfect living environment, including our atmosphere, for our good and that we would be wise to be attentive to it.

Furthermore, animal agriculture may be a causal factor in changing weather patterns. The number-one concern that we have is the role of deforestation, particularly of the precious Amazon rainforests, which are being destroyed at an alarming rate to raise livestock for beef. **In fact, animal agriculture is responsible for up to 91 percent of Amazon destruction.**[88] To increase the land available to raise farm animals in South America, one to two acres of rainforest are cleared every second.[89] It is known that the enormous size of the Amazon does affect weather worldwide and that deforestation of the rainforest impacts weather patterns.[90] Also, we learned that forest loss contributes to 25 percent of the world's greenhouse emissions.[91]

Additional impacts that our animal-based diets have on the environment are the contamination and reduction of clean water, and there are several reasons for this. Immense volumes of water resources are used at alarming rates to feed and slaughter animals for food. And to exacerbate the problem, animal waste runoff from these practices often contaminates waterways, affecting both human and animal life.

Oftentimes when we think about water shortages, we think about them occurring halfway around the world. But water scarcity is familiar to many in the United States, too. Most people don't know about the enormous water usage in animal agriculture and how it impacts us here at home. In fact, we were surprised to learn that California agriculture sends one hundred billion gallons of the state's water to Asia each year in the form of alfalfa.[92] Why would California support this practice when the state regularly experiences times of drought? The short answer is money. Asia is rapidly adopting the Western diet of animal-based foods, and alfalfa is the feed of choice for their factory farms. But alfalfa is one of the biggest water hogs there is. We don't believe that most Californians even know that this is happening to their precious water. So what's the solution? Perhaps California farmers and citizens would benefit more from keeping their water to grow plant crops intended for human consumption that do not require such large quantities of water.

An astonishing practice in animal agriculture is the use of enormous amounts of water to slaughter animals for human food—more than one hundred and thirty-two gallons per animal. That may not sound like a lot until you realize that more than nine billion animals are slaughtered for food in the US alone (2015), which comes to more than 1.2 trillion gallons of water used annually. Globally, seventy billion animals a year—nearly six million land animals every hour—are slaughtered worldwide.[93] That's a lot of water!

Lastly, one of the less known (albeit significant) effects of animal agriculture is runoff of animal feces into our lands and into our waterways: streams, lakes, and eventually oceans. In many parts of the world, this creates unsanitary water conditions for drinking, cooking, dishwashing, and bathing. In addition, this contaminated water runoff can cause algae to grow out of control in lakes and other bodies of water. This, in turn, affects our fish and other wildlife. The algae in these bodies of water cause the fish to suffocate, and the clean drinking water supply for wildlife is reduced.[94]

Toxic Burden

An additional environmental concern is the use of harsh pesticides and fertilizers. For example, we learned that some rice is grown in former cotton fields that were treated with the pesticide calcium arsenate (arsenic).[95] It has now been discovered that rice grown in these same fields contains potentially harmful levels of arsenic.[96] The latent effects of residual and accumulative arsenic in the human body from the consumption of this rice is being explored.[97] In light of the growing concerns about pesticides, we were happy to discover that alternative (and oftentimes more effective) farming practices exist. Traditional farming methods such as rotating crops, using cover crops, and resting land are sustainable techniques that can achieve many of the same goals as pesticides and fertilizers and provide better disease-resistant crops. In fact, the National Catholic Rural Conference encourages people in poor nations to use traditional farming methods to achieve better results.[98] A way to complement these traditional practices is to grow organic crops that use fewer and less harmful pesticides and fertilizers.

A Simpler Way

So what can be done to protect, preserve, and nourish our planet, or what Pope Francis calls "our common home," in a way that can benefit us and future generations? Perhaps you have heard that renewable energy is the answer. Or that taking fewer or shorter showers is the answer. Or that driving an electric car is the answer. Or that reducing home energy consumption is the answer. These actions might help, but we believe that there is a far greater, more efficient, less costly—and simpler—solution that diminishes harmful impacts to the environment and simultaneously benefits human health and promotes life in all of its forms. **A WFPB diet is that simpler solution.**

We may not have a full understanding about the impact that our decisions have on the environment and our long-term survival. However, we do know that meat and dairy require exponentially more water, land, and other resources to produce than most fruits and vegetables do. The production of cattle (raising, feeding, transporting, and slaughtering), combined with their waste run-off, is responsible for many serious ecological issues.[99] In contrast, plant foods, especially when organically and traditionally grown, do not cause the same widespread degradation of the environment. In addition to the health benefits, we believe that eating organic, whole, starch- and plant-based foods is the single most effective action that we can each take to reduce our human footprint on the Earth. The good news is that if every human reduced their animal consumption by even a small percentage, it would have a tremendous, positive effect on the environment.

The political issues sometimes muddy the waters when it comes to how we treat our planet, mostly because of the conflicting (and oftentimes costly) ways that are proposed to improve the situation. In other words, how we address this environmental threat is where things become complex and confusing, but it doesn't have to be complicated.

In the Native American tradition, there is a principle known as 7th Generation. This principle dates back more than a thousand years. The philosophy requires that every decision and choice take into account how the next seven generations will be affected by it. This way of life can provide a lot of valuable insight as we make our own decisions, particularly about the planet, and how our choices will affect future generations and the survival of the human race and animal wildlife.

you can't call yourself an environmentalist and still eat meat and dairy.
—James Cameron

Food for Thought:

1. What most surprised you about how the rich, animal-based Western diet impacts the environment?
2. If you knew that making a simple change from eating meat to eating beans would make a big impact for the environment, would you be willing to make that change?
3. Do you believe that we have a responsibility to live in such a way as to help ensure that people everywhere have clean water to drink and healthy food to eat?
4. Do you believe that the Church and the Christian faithful have a moral obligation to help protect the Earth?

CHAPTER 5

ANIMALS

L ife Seed: The choices that we make about how to treat animals, along with for which purposes we assign them, affect human life in innumerable, sobering, and consequential ways. We have a moral obligation to understand the choices that we make with regard to animals and how those choices impact human life.

> Father, we praise you with all your creatures.
> They came forth from your all-powerful hand;
> they are yours, filled with your presence and your tender love.
> Praise be to you!
> —Pope Francis, *Laudato Si*

Most people would say that they have an appreciation for animals. Many of us love our dogs, cats, fish, and other pets. We enjoy watching the birds, deer, bunnies, and other critters in our backyards. We love seeing documentaries about wolves and grizzly bears. Some of us even take vacations to witness the strength, beauty, and speed of lions, tigers, and gazelles, as well as the majesty of elephants and giraffes. The warm, positive feelings that we have toward these wondrous animals point to our innate connection to all of God's creatures. We naturally flinch and feel sadness when we see them hurt, in pain, or being mistreated.

The Harsh Reality

When we think of animal cruelty, we tend to think of isolated cases related to dogs and cats perpetrated by heartless owners or criminals. Animal cruelty is something that most of us cannot imagine participating in or condoning. But the hidden reality is that we do—even if unwittingly—every time we eat an animal-based food or purchase many other animal-based, non-food products like leather, fur, wool, makeup, supplements, and many other everyday household products. Cruel and systematic abuse is the **legal and prescribed norm** of our factory farm food system from which most of our animal-based foods come. Animals that are grown for food are considered commodities (hence the term "livestock") and have little to no protection, unlike our household pets. Most would be shocked to learn about the unrelenting harshness and routine inhumane practices of this callous and brutal factory farm industry.

READER ALERT: It may be hard to believe (and difficult to read below), but some common factory farm practices are the following:

Chickens:
Male baby chicks cannot produce eggs, so they are either ground up alive or tossed alive into large garbage

bags, which are then sealed so that the chicks suffocate to death.

Chickens raised in crates can't move or turn around. Even those deemed "free range" have only a space smaller than a piece of paper to move.

Many chickens are pumped with large amounts of antibiotics and hormones so that their breasts grow so big that they cannot walk nor sustain the weight of their own bodies.

Some chickens raised in the United States are shipped to China (with no food or water) for slaughter and then shipped back for American consumption.

Pigs:

Male piglets are castrated and mutilated, and their tails are cut off without anesthesia or pain medicine.

Baby piglets who are sick or not growing sufficiently are often killed by having their heads slammed against the cement floor of the factory farms. These pigs are then used to make bacon.

Adult pigs are led into a "processing room." There they are strung up alive by one leg. They are dunked into a large vat of boiling hot water, then transferred to a spit where they are spiralized to remove their fur.

Cows:

Downer cows (ones that are too sick to stand) are shoveled up with backhoes and discarded alive into trash bins.

Many calves are taken from their mothers immediately after birth, leaving both baby and mother in a state of persistent and painful mourning...all so humans can drink the milk that the lactating mother is producing.

Other baby cows are fit with prong harnesses so that the mothers will reject the babies and prevent the babies from nursing.

Many male baby cows are put into veal crates immediately after birth, where they never receive their own mother's milk or see the light of day. Julia Child, the famed French chef, stopped cooking veal after going to a veal farm (as recounted by author John Robbins[100]).

Cows are repeatedly electrocuted in the head with stun guns, and they are then tied up by their feet and have their throats slit. However, many are not adequately stunned and are still aware of what's happening because of the fast pace of the factory farming system.

Cannulas (holes) are surgically fit into holes cut into the sides of cows, allowing farmers to analyze the digestive tracts in order to provide the most efficient feed. The cannulas keep the holes open to prevent them from healing over.

Sheep:
In Australia, sheep are sheered for wool and then sent by ship (with no water or food) to the Middle East, where they have their throats slits with no anesthesia whatsoever.

Sheep are sheered so quickly because of the pressure that workers are under to move at a fast pace. This often results in a brutal sheering. Little to no care is taken to how the wool is removed with the very sharp sheers. Their skin is often cut, gouged, and removed during this quick

process. Sheep are routinely beaten and punched in the head to keep them from squirming.
This is only a glimpse of the unthinkable acts that are thrust on the animals.

Animal abuse in factory farming quietly damages the human psyche.
—Mark Bittman, journalist and author[101]

It may be hard to reconcile these practices with our love for animals. It was really difficult for us to learn about them. Because of United States ag gag Laws (factory farm anti-whistleblower laws), most people are not even aware of many of these issues. For more on these and other factory farming practices, please refer to the organizations Mercy for Animals and Compassion over Killing, as well as the documentaries *Peaceable Kingdom* and *Earthlings*.

The Impact

The thinking man must oppose all cruel customs no matter how deeply rooted in tradition and surrounded by a halo. When we have a choice, we must avoid bringing torment and injury into the life of another, even the lowliest creature; to do so is to renounce our manhood and shoulder a guilt which nothing justifies.
—Albert Schweitzer, theologian, writer, philosopher, and physician

We were given responsibility to take care of God's creatures, and instead, they have been exploited in the cruelest ways. The *CCC* (#2416) tells us that we "owe them [animals] kindness." We believe that we need to look at these issues with open eyes to see if they are in line with our core values about life. The USCCB writes that we are to have respect for human life, "which extends to respect for all of creation."[102]

> God cannot look on "objectively" while his creatures suffer. To imagine him doing so is to imagine someone quite other than God.
> —Thomas Merton, Trappist monk[103]

Children are born with an innate sense of care and compassion for animals. We were raised with many pets ourselves…dogs, a cat, guinea pigs, fish, a turtle, and a frog. We still enjoy having pets today as adults. What we have noticed is that kids have to be taught *not to care* about an animal's well-being, including farm animals. We have heard of other people's experiences describing the endearing feelings that they had as children toward the farm animals that they raised. They then shared the sadness that they felt when they realized that the animals were going to be killed for their food or someone else's. This caused many of them internal conflict and painful memories. We are taught as Catholics that it is imperative to pay attention to and follow our conscience. The *CCC* (#344) states that there is a "solidarity among all creatures arising from the fact that all have the same Creator." This makes sense, and children understand this intuitively.

> If any kid ever realized what was involved in factory farming, they would never touch meat again.

—James Cromwell, actor who starred in the movie *Babe*

What we consume has a very powerful effect on us—physically, mentally, and spiritually. How, then, is it affecting us to consume animals that have died undeserved, unwanted, and violent deaths? How might that be reinforcing our own aggressive tendencies? People often say that if a child shows a pattern of abusing animals (or even abuses one animal), he or she might be suffering from some sort of psychological problem and is someone who may be prone to hurting other people as an adult.[104] However, millions of people who work in factory farms and slaughterhouses (where animals are routinely abused) are required to participate in the most inhumane treatment and slaughter of animals. We're not implying that these people will harm other humans as a result of their workplace conditions. But we are convinced that people, often undocumented workers, who participate in animal farming, do suffer at a deep, often unconscious, level from a great deal of anguish for their actions. In fact, we learned that people who work in factory farms are prone to, and often suffer from, post-traumatic stress disorder (PTSD) from the work that they do.[105] Unfortunately, these workers (particularly those who are in this country illegally) may feel trapped because it's one of the few jobs that they can get. We believe that it is not possible to kill another being, human or otherwise, and not suffer some internal conflict. (As a side note, *eating* animals also affects how we feel emotionally. There is a significant correlation between reduced incidence of depression and eliminating animal products from the diet. Dr. Michael Greger reports that moods can lift after only two weeks of removing animals-based foods.[106])

__The Tsunami is Building__

> ...when we do something to protect animals, this act has significance beyond just helping that animal. It is part of a larger restorative effort that mends our relationships with one another and God as well.
> —Reasa Currier, Strategic Initiatives Manager, Faith Outreach Program, Humane Society of United States[107]

The *CCC* (#2418) states that it "is contrary to human dignity to cause animals to suffer or die needlessly." We have laws that protect animals from *unnecessary* suffering. But the suffering that "food" animals endure is considered *necessary*. In reality, we learned that it is **not necessary** because we do not need to eat animals, nor their byproducts, for our health. It's just the opposite. As we discussed in the first and second chapters, an animal-based diet is at the root of many chronic illnesses and reproductive issues.

As we would expect, most Americans prefer to buy humanely raised animal-based foods, even if it means paying a little more.[108] This tells us that most people intuitively want the best for animals. Because of public awareness and outcry, some factory farming practices are changing. But the most humane practice is to adopt a plant-based diet. Many are now learning, as we did, that humans do not need to consume animals or use their byproducts to survive or even thrive.

We grew up eating animals like most people do. As strange as it seems to us now, the disparity between what we were eating and what it really entailed did not fully resonate until we were adults. Jennifer had a few particularly "in-your-face" experiences that she shares here:

At the time, I was eating a paleo diet and getting all of my "meat" from a local farmer. When our first order of beef was delivered, the farmer's wife said to me with sadness (about the cow that had been slaughtered), "He was such a good boy and climbed right up into the truck." I felt heartbroken and sick to my stomach as I looked at the hot steaming beef in the back of her truck. Then, one Sunday morning on the way to Mass, we passed the farm. Jokingly, my younger son said, "Mom, look at the cow out there. Are you going to kill him, too?" My son meant nothing by the comment, but the sudden realization of what I had been doing was like a dagger in my heart. I love animals, and I couldn't stand the thought that I was sending many of them to their deaths.

About a month later, right before Thanksgiving, I went to the farm to get some eggs. The farmer asked if I wanted any turkeys for Thanksgiving, and I ordered two. He led me to the barn to see the turkeys. Inside, I saw half a dozen beautiful turkeys running around. I was very upset as I drove down the farmer's long driveway and back home. When I cooked the turkeys for Thanksgiving a few weeks later, it was heart-wrenching for me. I had one small piece of turkey and wanted to cry.

After watching the documentary Forks over Knives *and having become familiar with the works of Dr. McDougall and others, we agreed that a WFPB diet is the healthiest diet there is and the way we wanted to eat.*

We would like to make a clear distinction between family farms and factory farms. We personally know local farmers who raise animals for their own food and treat these creatures with great love and care. Many of them find it difficult when the time comes to send them away to be butchered. We fully respect these farmers and their hard-working way of life. While it's still true that the eating of animals is not good for human health and that animals are clearly impacted, we are far more concerned with the methods employed by factory farms.

> A farm is a peculiar problem for a man who likes animals, because the fate of most livestock is that they are murdered by their benefactors. The creatures may live serenely, but they end violently, and the odor of doom hangs about them always.
> —E.B. White, author of the children's book, *Charlotte's Web*
> (Note: the majority of animals *used* in today's food production do NOT live serenely.)

Food for Thought:

1. *If you eat anima-based foods (meat, dairy, fish, and eggs), have you ever considered where your food comes from or how it is produced? Is it important to you to know?*
2. *After reading about how animals are "produced" for human consumption, has it impacted how you think/feel about food?*
3. *Can you remember a time in your life (perhaps as a child) when you questioned the logic of eating animals?*
4. *Do you believe that humans have a moral responsibility to care for animals (not just pets) and to ensure that they are not mistreated?*
5. *Do you think the ways in which we "produce" animals for food lines up with what God intended when He gave us dominion over them?*
6. *Do you think that the Church and the faithful have a responsibility toward God's non-human animals?*

Part II
Our Response

CHAPTER 6

BRIDGING THE POLITICAL DIVIDE

Not left. Not right. Catholic!
—The Good News Letter

For far too long, political divides have prevented people from coming together on very important life issues—deeply connected issues. Those who would typically care for animal welfare and try to prevent food from being genetically modified are often the very same people who advocate for abortion, the death penalty, euthanasia, cloning, and genetically modifying humans. And those who are traditional, pro-life supporters often do not embrace protective measures for the environment or animals. Yet all of life is sacred and comes from God. Yes, humans come first in the order of things, but creation is not a zero-sum game. We do not need to minimize the value of the environment and animals to put humans first because what is good (the best) for the environment, animals, crops, and the planet is also the best for humans. The beautiful part is that we do not need to take opposite sides… it is all the same side! What is good for one truly is good for all. We may not find political figures who are willing to span the divide, but we, the people, can build a bridge ourselves. We can all make choices and purchases that get us closer to embracing life in all of its forms (and moving away from a culture of death).

Every issue is at stake and connected to the other. For instance, it may be surprising to know that we could take a big step toward smaller government if we made WFPB food choices. Here's why: skyrocketing health-care costs (from chronic diseases) that bankrupt individuals and nations would be dramatically reduced. Billions in funding research to find the "cures" for cancer, diabetes, and heart disease, among others, could also be drastically reduced. (For many of these lifestyle diseases, we already have the primary ingredient for the cures—our food.) Millions in lost wages and productivity would vanish from expenses connected to food-related illnesses that we get from eating animals. Billions more would be saved by reducing expenditures related to social security disability, prescription medication subsidies, water treatment for animal waste, and research into combating climate change, among others. We are not saying that all of these problems would disappear, but they could be dramatically improved and therefore be far more manageable. As things stand now, the system is buckling under the weight of all of these economic, civil, and societal problems.

If we want smaller government, lower taxes, fewer subsidies, better health-care insurance coverage for less money, real solutions to feed the hungry, and good health for everyone, then adopting a whole food, starch- and plant-based, oil-free diet *is once again the single most effective and simple answer*. What we are proposing transcends the political divide because whatever the issue, the food can be a huge part of the solution. We explore here a few points of commonality that we believe already exist among Americans and describe how a plant-based diet can further bridge those areas to benefit everyone.

1. **Full disclosure**: We, as Americans, desire transparency from our leaders. We believe that everyone wants (and has the right) to know the truth about our food and to understand how our food choices are impacting our health, our economy, our environment, the hungry, the animals, and our lives. Yet the institutions and systems that we ought to be able to trust have frequently—even intentionally—kept this information hidden from the public. Even when information about the food is made available or searched out, it is sometimes purposely distorted to mislead our citizens.

   We're not advocating that meat and dairy foods should somehow be outlawed. And we're not anti-farming. As we stated before, from our own experiences, we know that farmers are hard-working and dedicated folks. We simply want people to be able to make well-informed decisions about the foods that they consume, as well as how this food impacts their health and the world. And we want our trusted institutions to stop working in ways that are circular, counterproductive, deceptive, and misleading. We believe that we should be able to expect full disclosure about our food from all of our leaders (if they even *know* the truth). This, we believe, can become an area of unity for the benefit of all Americans.

   Fortunately, in the meantime, a number of organizations (including the PCRM and the Environmental Working Group) and documentaries (e.g., *Forks over Knives*; *PlantPure Nation*; *Earthlings*; *Cowspiracy*; *Food, Inc.;* and *Vegucated*) have done an excellent job of exposing the truth about our food and its implications for individuals, societies, animals, and our planet.

2. **Financial**: We Americans like to spend money, but there aren't many of us who enjoy paying more than we have to for something. We all like a good deal. Unfortunately, we are getting a raw deal when it comes to our food and how it affects our personal and national finances. As things stand now, we are not just paying for our food at the grocery store. We first pay for our food in taxes (up to 50 percent subsidies for the meat and dairy industries). We then pay for our food at the grocery stores. Next, we pay our healthcare premiums, which are enormously costly because of our current health-care crisis (as a result of the standard American diet). We then pay our doctors in co-pays and deductibles. We pay in lost work and productivity. And we pay with our lives.

   Because so many are unaware of the truth about our food and the corollary costs, Americans are spending exponentially more money for food than is necessary or just. As an antidote, if we, instead, chose to eliminate taxpayer subsidies to animal agriculture, unhealthy foods would naturally rise in price, leading people to less expensive and healthier options, such as starches. As market demand for healthier food options (organic plant-based food) increased, the prices would go down even further. Consumption of these healthier foods would then result in improved health outcomes. Subsequently, our health-care crisis would be greatly minimized; our health-care premiums would plummet; and we would live much healthier, happier, and more productive lives.
3. **Feeding**: As Americans, we love to give to those less fortunate. We have a long-standing history of generous giving to struggling nations. We want to know, though, that

the money and resources that we give (both personal and federal) are well spent and are making a difference. And to a certain degree, they are. Many more people around the world would be starving if it were not for the generosity of the United States and its citizens. However, because many of the food resources that we provide are animal based, we are not making as healthful or vast an impact as we could.

We suggest that there is one significant step that we can take to multiply the billions of US taxpayer dollars currently spent (annually) on humanitarian aid: *replace the animal-based foods that we currently provide to the hungry and poor with traditional starch- and other plant-based foods, which cost far less.* Further, providing these foods (and the funds to support them) would help curb disease in struggling nations. And as mentioned previously, some of the money could be spent to reintroduce local and sustainable farming programs that teach indigenous people how to grow their own food. This could provide valuable work skills and much-needed income for the poor, as well as a path toward food independence. Additionally, water-well assistance programs could be further expanded.

4. **Freedom**: The United States was founded on freedom, and most Americans want to keep it. All would acknowledge that freedom often comes with a human cost. Regardless of whether people support the just-war principle, most Americans support our soldiers and believe in the necessity of maintaining some kind of a military. We depend on the military to defend our freedom, and thanks to our bravest, we have enjoyed relative peace to this point.

Unfortunately, we learned that something *right now* is threatening our military and potentially our freedom. The

Pentagon reported that it is concerned about the rising obesity rates in the military. This shouldn't come as a surprise, given the American way of eating. According to a Mission Readiness report, almost 75 percent of Americans between the ages of seventeen and twenty-four years old are not eligible for military service for a variety of reasons, including obesity.[109] Overweight soldiers on active duty may cause risks in terms of health-care expenses and military readiness. The poor health of our soldiers is not only a threat to their own lives but is a serious national threat.

Having the ability to protect our country is a critical issue and one that needs to be addressed. One simple way is through nutrition. According to Rich Roll (a super-endurance athlete, best-selling author, and popular podcaster), some of our soldiers are indicating that they have an interest in a plant-based diet.[110] Perhaps our soldiers might individually consider the benefits of adopting Daniel's diet (Dan. 1:8–15). Daniel, the Old Testament prophet and soldier, and his friends ate only plant-based foods and were stronger and healthier than the king's other soldiers. This suggestion for our military men and women to adopt a plant-based diet is not to deprive them but instead to strengthen them and give them the best health and physical condition possible. We believe that the health and readiness of our soldiers is another issue on which many Americans can come together.

5. **Faith**: Many Americans of faith share important values. Issues of faith appear all over the political landscape, and so there is often disagreement, even between those who believe in God. But those of us raised in the Judeo-Christian faiths have some common Biblical texts, one of

which is Genesis—the first book of both the Torah and the Bible. In it, we are told that God created the Heavens and the Earth and all that lives on the Earth. He created the planet, the atmosphere, the vegetation, the animals, and humankind. And He declared it all very good. Most agree, to some extent, that everything that God created has and deserves some degree of dignity. The good news is that a plant-based diet inherently dignifies all that God created, particularly human life.

Politics that interfere with the truth about our food shouldn't be allowed to threaten the health of our citizens or the fitness and readiness of our soldiers. We deserve better as Americans and as sons and daughters of God. We believe that better is possible. A groundswell of awareness and action is already motivating and helping people to change and transition to a WFPB way of eating. Our elected officials would be wise to acknowledge the importance of a whole food, starch- and plant-based diet and to understand how it can improve many of the world's most pressing issues. The great news is you don't have to be affiliated with a particular political party to eat this way.

Food for Thought:

1. *Have you noticed how wide is the chasm between our political parties and their ideologies when it comes to issues of life?*
2. *Prior to reading this book, did you know that meat and dairy were heavily subsidized by the federal government?*
3. *It is estimated that a typical restaurant hamburger would cost upward of $50.00 without government subsidies. If your animal-based food costs went up because the government stopped*

subsidizing meat and dairy, would that influence your food choices?
4. *Had you ever thought about the connection between our animal-based diets and the size of the federal government?*
5. *Does it concern you that our military readiness is at risk due, in part, to obesity?*
6. *Do you believe that our citizens and military personnel deserve to know the truth from institutional and governmental advisors about our food?*
7. *How else might widespread adoption of a plant-based diet bridge our political divide?*

CHAPTER 7

THE CHURCH'S ROLE

> ...and you will know the truth, and the truth will set you free.
> —John 8:32

The Catholic Church is the church of faith and reason. Faith and reason can (and does) inform us of the gravity of the choices that we make, including when it comes to what we eat. The Church can take a world-leading role by considering and propagating the validity and value of how a WFPB diet can significantly and positively impact much of what ails humanity and how it can put us back in touch with what God has intended for the world. Many of the saints of old knew the health benefits and spiritual efficacy of temperance, which often included not consuming animals. (For more on the subject, we highly recommend reading *Vegetarian Christian Saints*.[111])

Catholic author and speaker Mathew Kelly often encourages us to "Become the-Best-Version-of-Yourself." We believe that making informed and better food choices can help us all to become a better version of ourselves and can help us to make a better version of our world. A plant-based lifestyle takes all aspects of life into account and puts humans in harmony with each other, with all of creation, and with Catholic pro-life principles. We can look to the cardinal virtues (prudence, justice, fortitude, temperance) and the theological virtues (faith, hope, charity) to inform and guide us about all of life, including our food choices.

> Easy choices, hard life. Hard choices, easy life.
> —Jerzy Gregorek, author of *The Happy Body*

The Catholic Church has often led the way in these matters illuminating from the beginning that everything was created by God and must be treated with dignity and respect, particularly human life. The Church is the most outspoken pro-life institution in the world. Happily, many Catholics and other Christian and non-Christian religious traditions are beginning to embrace the idea that the ways in which we treat creation and its creatures, human and non-human alike, are deeply moral issues and must be considered very carefully. We believe that the Church should be proclaiming the Good News and the world in all truth, including about how the food that we purchase and consume can lead to life (and death) in its many forms.

> Yet even if Revelation [in Jesus Christ] is already complete, it has not been made completely explicit; it remains for Christian faith gradually to grasp its full significance.
> —*Catechism of the Catholic Church,* #66

Food for Thought:

1. *How does a plant-based diet align with the cardinal virtues? How can I apply the cardinal virtues to my own relationship with food?*

Prudence

Justice

Fortitude

Temperance

2. *How does a plant-based diet align with the theological virtues? How can I apply the theological virtues to my own relationship with food?*

Faith

Hope

Charity

CHAPTER 8

CHANGE THE FOOD, CHANGE THE WORLD

> To whom much is given, much is expected.
> —Luke 12:48

What God created is good—He has told us so. And as mentioned earlier in the book, Sacred Scripture clearly indicates that humans inherited the Earth from God and have been given dominion over it. What an awesome privilege and responsibility we have as stewards. We can continually learn how to better care lovingly and gently for what has been entrusted to us by our Lord, the Good King.

> For what can be known about God is evident to them, because God made it evident to them. Ever since the creation of the world, his invisible attributes of eternal power and divinity have been able to be understood and perceived in what he has made.
> —Rom. 1:19–20

Unfortunately, the upside-down world that we live in is one that oftentimes doesn't seem to know or care about God or His creation.

As a consequence of turning away from God, of poor stewardship, and the resulting culture of death, our world is riddled with disease of all kinds: hunger, thirst, illness, obesity, poverty (and other serious economic problems), greed, violence, psychological problems, and erratic weather patterns, among others. None of us is immune. The havoc wrought in our bodies, in our minds, and on our planet are, at least in part, a result of seemingly "harmless" food choices. Animal-based foods and processed foods are harming us and depleting and destroying our natural resources—and many people don't even realize it. Genetically modified foods are tampering with God's perfect creation, and we don't know where this will lead. Man-made attempts to make a better world using human "solutions" (such as abortion, doctor-assisted suicide, and medical interventions that can cause a cascade of complications) are often counter to God's perfect ways (Isa. 55:8–9). Turning back to God, along with being mindful of everything that we do, can help us to better avoid unintended consequences.

To see God in one thing is to see Him in all things.
—Ignatian spirituality

Through our experiences and research, we began to recognize that when we *choose* to eat animals and their by-products, we are *choosing* (almost always *unintentionally*) to be out of balance, to contaminate our bodies, to overlook the immense suffering of people and animals around the world, to devastate nature, and to continue funding industries and ideas that are not always in our best interests. The domino effect of our food choices is staggering. We learned that we are *choosing* to use precious land for animals that could be used to grow crops to feed the hungry. We are *choosing* to deny clean water to the thirsty, as scarce supplies of clean water are contaminated by animal waste. We are *choosing* illness, as all of the best science and data unequivocally points to and concludes that consuming animals is one of the largest determiners of disease initiation and promotion. We are *choosing* to devastate our naturally beautiful habitats by overfishing our oceans and destroying the irreplaceable rainforests. We are *choosing* to compromise the health of our planet and atmosphere, as the production of meat and dairy is the number-one factor in greenhouse gas emissions. We are *choosing* hefty economic burdens because chronic diseases caused by our animal-based diets require expensive, drastic procedures and result in crushing health-care costs. The deleterious effects of *choosing* to purchase, eat, and consume animal-based products is endless.

Since this information is largely hidden from us, sometimes intentionally, most people don't even realize the impact that our food choices have on each and every one of us. When it comes to the impact that our food has on humans, the animals, and the Earth, the desire for money and power has often replaced the Golden Rule. Our children, hospital patients, the poor, and the public at large have been—and continue to be—victims of the misinformation and disinformation about the food and how it relates to every life issue. When we learned the truth, we were shocked. We believe that righteous anger was warranted and still is. Our anger was the impetus for our writing this book.

The good news (as you've read throughout this book) is that we have the ability to turn things around. We have more control that we may realize! When we embrace truth, we are empowered to make choices that benefit ourselves and our loved ones. When we *choose* to eat organic fruits, vegetables, and starches, we are *choosing* wholesome foods (and thus *choosing* to feel good and to be healthy). We are *choosing* to be kind and compassionate stewards of our Earth. We are *choosing* to take responsibility for ourselves and to consider those who are less fortunate. We are *choosing* to treat our bodies as temples of the Holy Spirit.

> I have set before you life and death, the blessing and the curse. Choose life, then, that you and your descendants may live.
> —Deut. 30:19

Food is so foundational to who we are. It has the ability to nourish us. It is the central element around which we gather together in communion and fellowship. It impacts every part of our human existence. And our choices about it generate consequences (good or bad) for all of creation. We have the opportunity to be completely "transformed by the renewing of our minds" (Rom. 12:2) with this information. We are so grateful that we were eventually awakened to the beautiful and holy interconnectedness of God, of our food, and of the state of our world.

> Begin with the beautiful, which leads to the good, which leads to the truth.
> —Bishop Robert Barron, auxiliary bishop for the Archdiocese of Los Angeles and founder of Word on Fire Catholic Ministries

We thank you, our readers, for staying with us as we put forth the holy connections between food and life issues: human health, reproduction, the poor and the hungry, the environment, and animals. Throughout the book, we have offered suggestions for fostering a culture of life through our food choices, and we maintain that real continued changes are possible but that they will only come through individuals who decide to make the personal choice, based on faith and reason (not on laws or mandates), to adopt a WFPB diet. We believe that if we change the food, we will change the world.

> The truth does not change according to our ability to stomach it.
> —Flannery O'Connor, American writer, essayist, and novelist

Food for Thought:

1. *Do you believe that humans have a responsibility for the wellbeing of other people, the Earth, and animals? If so, what does responsibility toward each look like? How do those responsibilities differ?*
2. *After reading this book, do you see a holy interconnectedness between God, pro-life issues, and the foods that we eat?*
3. *Do you believe that by changing our food, we can change the world?*
4. *How will you respond?*

Part III
Common Objections

CHAPTER 9

Common Objections and Our Responses

1) Vegans eat tofu, kale, and salads. I don't like those foods, so there is no way that I could be vegan.
We rarely eat tofu. Tofu can be, but is not typically, the center of a WFPB diet. Our personal diets consist mostly of starches, fruits, and other vegetables. We eat foods like potatoes, rice, other whole grains, corn, legumes, non-starchy vegetables, and a wide variety of luscious fruit. We do eat kale because we have found that kale added to many dishes, such as steel-cut oats and soups, is actually quite delicious. However, kale is not necessary for adopting a healthy vegan diet, either. We love salads and eat them often, but we don't eat them exclusively or as the center of our meals.

2) Vegan diets are just for hippies and hipsters.
Unfortunately, vegans have often been misunderstood and perceived as living on the fringe. For this reason, we shied away from identifying ourselves as vegans until we realized that being vegan is the most pro-life way to live. The new face of veganism is becoming more mainstream now than ever. There are many doctors, endurance athletes, professional ball players, celebrities, and politicians

who have learned the truth about the food and have adopted this way of eating for the reasons that we stated in the book. Though not well known, people from all walks of life—conservatives, liberals, people from all religions and regions—have already adopted the WFPB way of eating. Their reasons are varied, but health is among the top reasons.

3) I know some vegans who don't look very healthy, are overweight, and eat foods that I know are unhealthy.
We know about some of those people, too. Usually, they are vegetarians who consume dairy products, or they are vegans who eat large quantities of processed, oil-filled vegan junk foods. People who eat in these ways may have adopted their dietary habits for reasons other than health, or they think it's healthier than eating animal-based foods. They do not understand the negative health implications of eating vegan foods that are not whole, plant-based, and oil-free. These poorer eating habits can result in excess body weight and disease.

4) Vegans seem to care more about animals than people. And at times, they elevate animals to the status of humans.
Some people do seem to care more about animals than people. While the treatment of animals is very important, and we believe that they should be cared for, this does not mean that animals take the place of, or come before, human life. People have multiple reasons for adopting a WFPB diet, and more and more people are adopting it for health reasons. Once people come to understand that eating animals is not necessary for health (and, in fact, is detrimental to health), they begin to learn more about the many other positive benefits of eating a plant-based diet. These benefits include the sparing of billions of animals from being unnaturally

and intensively bred, treated poorly, tortured, and killed. Animals are very vulnerable and depend on us for care and compassion.

5) There is not enough food to feed the world. We need animals, genetically modified organisms (GMOs), and pesticides to meet the world's hunger crisis. To further solve the problem, we also need to expand worldwide population control measures like abortion and euthanasia.

GMOs and pesticides: Organic crops grown in accord with God's natural laws can produce equivalent (or greater) harvests and are more drought resistant than genetically modified, pesticide-laden crops.[112] In the long run, growing GMO crops and using harmful pesticides actually work against the solution to providing healthy food to the hungry. Fortunately, organizations like Catholic Relief Services are helping populations to grow foods with traditional farming methods.[113]

We are alarmed that there are a few large companies that produce and own the majority of GMO seeds. The fruits and vegetables of these seeds often do not produce seeds; therefore, these crops cannot produce additional food. This gives a few large companies more and more control of our seed supply.

Animals: Raising, feeding, watering, and producing animals for food is actually much less efficient than producing and growing crops for people. And to top it off, eating animals is dangerous to human health. Potatoes, beans, corn, rice (and other whole grains), vegetables, and fruits can feed whole populations—with perfect nutrition. According to Dr. Campbell, Dr. McDougall, Dr. Esselstyn, and other health and nutrition experts, people can healthfully thrive on these foods for their entire lives. In addition, these foods can be very inexpensive and affordable.

Population control: As previously discussed, more than 50 percent of all land in the world is used for animal agriculture. If we used that land for people and for plant-based food crops, we would be better able to feed the world. This might help to prevent people from considering ungodly means of controlling the population (e.g., contraceptives, abortion, euthanasia, and limiting the number of children that a family can bear).

6) God put animals on the Earth for us to eat.
We can gather from the creation narrative in the Bible (Gen. 1:29) that the first humans ate a diet of plant-based foods. However, as previously highlighted, the Biblical commentary on the same verse stated that "due to the propensity of humans to sin, God allowed humans to eat animals." Humans also have the propensity to allow their anger to get the best of them, and some people even kill other humans as a result. But does that mean that we should give in to our human imperfections? God has given every person free will and allows us to eat animals. However, in the words of Saint Paul, "All things are permissible, but not all things are beneficial" (1 Cor. 10:23). Given all that we learned about achieving and maintaining good health by eating a whole food, plant-based, oil-free diet, we came to the conclusion that we could make no other choice than to eliminate all animal products from our diet.

7) God has given us dominion over the animals (Gen. 1:26); therefore, we can do what we want with them.
The real definition of dominion reveals care and responsibility. Why would we treat the animals and the Earth with such disdain, harm, cruelty, and disrespect, especially when we have better, kinder, and healthier options?

8) Jesus said, "It is not what enters one's mouth that defiles that person; but what comes out of the mouth is what defiles one" (Matt. 15:11).

Jesus, we believe, was trying to communicate to His listeners that the Mosaic dietary laws do not make a person righteous. Instead, He was helping them to understand that our loving posture toward God and our neighbors is much more important than following specific dietary laws, which avail nothing. We agree completely. And while we recognize (and are grateful) that God has given us free will, has lifted the Mosaic dietary restrictions, and has *allowed* the eating of animals, we also understand that it is neither necessary nor healthy.

9) What would happen to the extra animals?

We wouldn't have excess animals because a worldwide transition to a plant-based diet would happen very gradually. Most farm animals are bred in factory farms specifically for the purpose of becoming food. The intensive breeding of billions of animals would be eliminated with the widespread adoption of a plant-based diet. Therefore, we wouldn't have cows, chickens, and pigs running through US city streets (as some have suggested), just as we don't have them doing that now.

10) We are carnivores. We were meant to eat meat.

We are not carnivores. Our teeth and our intestinal tracts attest to this. Our human teeth, in fact, are the same shape as other herbivores. Human intestinal tracts are long and winding. Our digestion is slow for the purpose of pulling out important nutrients from our food. Fiber is important for daily elimination and is only found in plant-based foods.[114]

11) We need to eat animals to maintain good health. Many doctors recommend eating lean meats and low-fat dairy (at least in limited quantities) for protein, iron, B-12, calcium, amino acids, and other nutrients.

Doctor recommendations: Traditionally, physicians have received about one to two hours of nutrition education, if that, during their schooling and interning years. As the introduction and expansion of nutrition education for medical professionals increases, the advice that doctors give to their patients is beginning to change. As mentioned earlier, the Academy of Nutrition and Dietetics (AND)—the largest organization of food and nutrition professionals—now considers the vegan diet to be one of the healthiest way to eat.[115] According to the association's website, AND represents over one hundred thousand credentialed practitioners. These professionals play a critical role in influencing our nation's food choices.

Protein, calcium, and iron: Protein, calcium, and iron are most ideally consumed by humans in the form of plant-based foods, such as potatoes, beans, corn, grains, leafy greens, and other vegetables.[116] In fact, most people consume too much protein and calcium in the form of animal-based foods and protein drinks, which are very hard on the kidneys and other organs.[117] These animal-based products are also laden with artery-clogging fats, which doctors generally do not recommend. Further, Dr. T. Colin Campbell's *The China Study* reveals that cancer can be turned on and off by increasing consumption (to 20 percent animal protein) or reducing consumption (to 5 percent animal protein), respectively.[118]

A varied plant-based diet containing sufficient calories does not come with the same cancer risks and adequately meets the United States recommended daily allowance (RDA) of protein at 8–10 percent of calories of food.[119] In addition, the consumption of starchy, vegetable-based protein consistently produces higher satiety levels than the consumption of animal-based proteins.[120]

Vitamin B-12: Vitamin B-12 is the one supplement that vegans do need to take. It is "produced by bacteria, not animals or plants," according to Dr. Sofia Pineda Ochoa. She explains that Vitamin B-12 is often found in manure, which contains a lot of bacteria, and says that B-12 is found in animal-based foods because farm animals often live in manure-laden environments and are even fed manure.[121] Thus, people who eat animals do get a little B-12. However, Dr. Neal Barnard, the founder of PCRM, says that even people who consume animal products need to take a B-12 supplement because most people are not getting enough.[122] Most vegans are not exposed to the bacteria via manure (because foods are usually washed); therefore, many doctors recommend a vitamin B-12 supplement for people who follow a plant-based diet.

Amino acids: It is often mistakenly taught that those who follow a plant-based diet need to combine foods in order to get all of the essential amino acids. However, the person who made the food-combining myth popular has recanted her original, erroneous statement. Plant-based foods provide complete and perfect nutrition for the human body.[123]

12) The United States government food guidelines recommend eating meat, dairy, fish, and egg products.
While it is true that our government recommends eating meat, dairy, fish, and eggs as part of the MyFood Plate program, those recommendations are inching toward a more plant-centric diet rich in nutrients. However, there are very powerful lobbyists in our country who have a vested interest in protecting the long-held

and popular belief that meat and other animal-based foods are the best protein sources for humans. They have spent years misleading and influencing government leaders to support their agendas. Any attempts to reduce or eliminate animal-based food products from US government food guidelines have been met with great resistance. In the documentary *PlantPure Nation*, numerous examples of this pushback are well illustrated. Despite US government guidelines, the World Health Organization and the United Nations recommend a plant-based diet for the purposes of health, climate, and meeting the world's food needs.[124]

In addition, there are now some foreign leaders advocating plant-based diets for their citizens. For example, the mayor of Turin, Italy, has encouraged the whole town to go vegetarian (and even vegan) to protect human health, the environment, and animal welfare.[125] And the former president of Ireland is now urging upcoming leaders to go vegan.[126] Further, the governor-general of New Zealand, who is in charge of the Royal Guard of Honor, is also vegan.[127]

In many areas of China, where traditional plant-based diets were customarily eaten, the people were healthy and trim, and they rarely experienced chronic illnesses like cancer, heart disease, and diabetes.[128] Now that the Chinese have adopted the standard American diet, chronic health problems, like those in Western nations, are becoming increasingly prevalent. In the last thirty-five years, the average Chinese citizen has increased meat consumption by more than one hundred pounds per year, explaining the increase in disease. As a result, the Chinese government has charted a plan to cut the country's meat consumption by half to substantially reduce its greenhouse gas emissions and to curb its spike in obesity and diabetes.[129] The country's leaders have also realized that its citizens' appetite for animal-based foods is unsustainable, given current world resources.

13) What would our meat and dairy farmers do for income if everyone stopped eating animal-based foods?
We have given much thought to the question of how meat and dairy farmers could make a living. If we retained government food subsidies, they could be redirected from animal-based farming to farmers willing to transition to plant-based farming, ideally organic. We would strongly support retaining subsidies for this purpose. As we previously mentioned, many meat and dairy farmers currently receive large government subsidies—thirty-eight *billion* dollars a year—while plant-based food farmers, on the other hand, receive just seventeen *million* dollars a year.[130] We recognize that a transition from animal-based farming to plant-based farming would take time, but even incremental steps would help in many ways. This transition would provide additional benefits: help to feed our world's population, cut down on environmental waste, and conserve natural resources.

While it might seem harsh at first blush to eliminate animal-based food subsidies, all industries must evolve as we learn new information. Innovation and creativity are the engines that made—and continue to make—America the most prosperous nation on Earth. It is possible in this agricultural sector to evolve beyond current practices for the good of all, including the farmers. Should we have continued to support tobacco companies in the face of overwhelming scientific evidence that smoking kills? Of course not! But despite the proof of the harmful effects of smoking, the tobacco and cigarette lobbyists continued to promote it. Fortunately, the evidence became so overwhelmingly clear about the deleterious health implications of smoking—and our government was willing to warn the public and change policies—that much of the public quit this deadly habit. Similarly, we are now faced with overwhelming scientific evidence implicating animal-based foods in disease initiation and progression. What will we choose to do? (We vote for appointing Dr. John McDougall as surgeon general!)

> It took more than 7,000 studies, and the death of countless smokers before the first Surgeon General report against smoking was finally released. Another mountain of evidence exists today for healthier eating, but much of society has yet to catch up to the science.
> —Dr. Michael Greger[131]

14) Adopting a WFPB diet means that all of my holiday meals and traditions will be ruined.
Turkey, ham, and other meats tend to be at the center of American holiday meal tables. But in truth, most of the foods on our holiday tables are plant-based side items: sweet potatoes, mashed potatoes, cranberry, green beans, glazed carrots, stuffing, corn, squash, wild rice, and mushroom gravy. And dessert usually includes pumpkin and apple pies. Every single one of these side dishes and desserts can be made deliciously without a single animal-based ingredient. For special occasions like holidays, delicious meat replacements (though not oil-free) like Gardein, Field Roast, Tofurkey, and Trader Joe's Breaded Turkey-less Roast are available. Additionally, Earth Balance vegan butter and Daiya vegan cheeses (also not oil-free) can be used for transitioning to a plant-based diet.

15) Feeding a vegan diet to babies is unhealthy and can even kill them.
In truth, a well-planned vegan diet containing *sufficient calories and vitamins* is a very healthy diet to feed to babies (once they are weaned from the mother's milk), toddlers, and children of all ages. If problems occur in young children who are fed vegan diets, they do not occur as a result of the vegan diet, per se. Rather, problems arise only when the child is being fed a diet insufficient in calories and nutrition, which results in malnutrition. Thus, adequate calories and proper nutrients are the keys to safely raising healthy children on a plant-based diet.[132] As with any child, regular healthy-baby check-ups are critical!

16) There is no conclusive evidence that genetically modified organisms (GMOs) are harmful to human health.
We don't believe that enough is known about GMOs and their long-term effects on the human body to determine if they are healthy or safe. Some GMO seeds are actually filled with pesticides so that the plants themselves will be able to stave off pests. These chemicals were created to affect the pests' nervous systems. If we, as humans, consume ever-greater amounts of these pesticides because we are encouraging people to eat large amounts of fruits and vegetables, how can we be sure that these pesticides are not affecting *our* nervous systems? It may be that consuming the pesticides in small amounts has a negligible effect. But we don't yet know what the cumulative effect of eating them is, and we don't know how these chemicals react with other chemicals we put into our bodies, namely pharmaceutical drugs. We are concerned about the unknown future impact of these seeds and chemicals on human health and on our food supply.

Another concerning trend is that many people in the United States have found that they have become sensitive to gluten. However, some have reported that when they go to European countries, they are able to eat breads and pasta with no problem. What accounts for this anecdotal phenomenon? We wonder if it is possible that this is because European countries do not allow GMO crops to be grown in their countries. In addition, from personal experience, we are not able to eat corn grown in this country unless it is organic (non-GMO), or we experience symptoms.

17) Organic foods are not worth the extra money.
We believe that, while organic foods can be more expensive, the health and safety benefits are worth it. Organic foods, by law, cannot contain GMOs, nor can they be treated with the harshest chemical pesticides. It is estimated by the Environmental Protection Agency that up to twenty thousand farmers and their families get pesticide poisoning each year.[133] People who spread these chemicals often wear hazardous material (hazmat) suits. This fact alone should raise red flags about the safety of consuming food treated with these chemicals. We don't know what the effect might be of these chemicals on the workers who pick the foods. As noted earlier, organic crops, fertilizers, and pesticides have, at times, been shown to be just as effective, if not more effective, in food production without potential harmful side effects. In addition, studies have found that organic, plant-based foods are more nutritious than their conventional counterparts.[134]

18) I live by the principle of "all things in moderation."
"All things in moderation" didn't work for us as a guiding principle. Moderation in "healthy" oils turned out to be counterproductive. Paula's cholesterol levels did not go down while she was consuming

these so-called "healthy" oils. In fact, they shot up with a moderate intake of these oils (and dropped seventy-nine points after eliminating them again). Also, Jennifer's weight increased with a moderate amount of fat intake from these same "healthy" oils. Further, the amounts of animal-based foods recommended in medical and governmental guidelines didn't make us healthy.

19) I've been told that I need to eat healthy fats.
We don't need to worry that we won't get any fat if we switch to a plant-based, oil-free diet because most plant foods contain some fat. People who choose to eat higher-fat plant foods, such as nuts and avocados, should eat them as whole foods. However, most people consume fats in the form of free (extracted) oils—olive, coconut, safflower, nut, etc. Despite popular claims, recent studies find that these oils are not very good for us. Dr. Gabe Mirkin, in one of his Weekly eZine articles, reported that a Swedish study demonstrated that saturated fats from plants increase diabetes risk. Dr. Mirkin's advice is to "restrict all foods high in saturated fats, whether from plant or animal sources."[135] Drs. John McDougall and Caldwell Esselstyn agree and further recommend avoiding *all added oils*, saturated or not.[136]

20) Jesus ate fish. Why shouldn't we?
There are multiple reasons why one might not want to eat fish: (1) Heavy metals and prescription medicines have been detected in some oceans and waterways; (2) antibiotics are used in fish farming; (3) overfishing causes depletion and extinction of marine life;[137] and (4) eating fish is not necessary and is, in fact, detrimental to human health. Thus, there doesn't appear to be any good reason to eat fish.

21) I don't believe in, nor do I care about, the issues you brought up in this book. I want to eat meat, dairy, fish, eggs, and processed junk food.
If you want to eat meat, dairy, fish, eggs, and processed junk food, then you certainly may. We are not advocating any new "food laws," whether religious or political. We are simply providing the most up-to-date information so that people can make wise food choices based on faith and reason.

22) I want to adopt a WFPB diet, but my family and/or friends don't support me.
There are many plant-based communities online. We feel confident that you will receive all of the support and emotional air that you need to pursue your plant-based lifestyle and succeed. You will be a great witness to those around you.

23) Okay, you've sold me on the idea of a whole food, plant-based, oil-free diet! What do I do now?
We are so happy for you! Get ready, because it's coming…a happier, healthier you. Check out some of our favorite books, documentaries, websites, and more on the "Our Favorite Resources" page in the next of section of this book.

Food for Thought:

1. *What other objections, questions, or concerns do you have about adopting a WFPB diet?*
2. *Do you know anyone who eats a vegan diet? What is your impression of him/her? Does it help or hinder your desire to consider a WFPB diet?*

3. *How difficult do you think that it would be to adopt a WFPB diet? What do you perceive might be some of the difficulties?*
4. *How would your holidays and other traditions be affected if you/your family eliminated animal-based foods from the menu? What are some of your favorite holiday foods? How might they be adapted to be whole food and plant-based?*
5. *What are some of your favorite foods? What foods could you substitute to adapt recipes to replace animal-based foods? (Examples include meat-based chili to bean-based chili, meat- and dairy-based lasagna to vegetable lasagna, and meat and dairy pizza to veggie pizza without cheese.)*

ABOUT THE AUTHORS

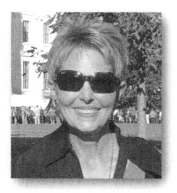 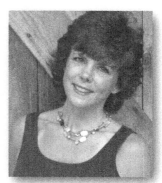

Paula B. Sandin and Jennifer S. Adams suffered for years from illnesses their doctors deemed incurable. They transformed their health through food choices and reawakened their faith through conversion to Catholicism. Today they operate A Litttle Light, an online T-shirt shop providing inspirational messages about God and healthy living. Originally from the Washington, DC, area, they now live in Huntsville, AL, and try to live out their Catholic faith to make a difference in the lives of everyone with whom they interact.

OUR FAVORITE RESOURCES

Books
Diet for a New America, by John Robbins
For Love of Animals, by Charlie Camosy
How Not To Die, by Dr. Michael Greger
Engine 2 Diet, by Rip Esselstyn
Meatanomics, by David Robinson Simon
Plant-Strong, by Rip Esselstyn
Prevent and Reverse Heart Disease, by Caldwell Esselstyn, Jr.
The China Study, by Dr. T. Colin Campbell and Dr. Thomas M. Campbell
The Pleasure Trap, by Dr. Douglas Lisle and Dr. Alan Goldhamer
The Starch Solution, by Dr. John McDougall
Whole, by T. Colin Campbell, with Howard Jacobson

Cookbooks
Forks over Knives Cookbook, by Del Sroufe and Isa Chandra Moskowitz
Plant-Strong (recipes in Rip Esselstyn's book)
Prevent and Reverse Heart Disease Cookbook: Over 125 Delicious, Life-Changing, Plant-Based Recipes, by Ann C. Esselstyn and Jane Esselstyn
The Starch Solution (recipes in Dr. John McDougall's book)

Documentaries
Cowspiracy
Earthlings
Escape Fire
Food Chains
Food, Inc.

Forks over Knives
Living on One Dollar A Day
Peaceable Kingdom: The Journey Home
PlantPure Nation
Vegucated
What the Health

Websites
Cooking with Plants (cookingwithplants.com)
Dr. McDougall's Health & Medical Center (drmcdougall.com)
Feasting on Fruit (feastingonfruit.com)
Forks over Knives (forksoverknives.com)
Fully Raw (fullyraw.com)
Happy Herbivore (happyherbivore.com)
Nutrition Facts (nutritionfacts.org)
Oh She Glows (ohsheglows.com)
Ordinary Vegan (ordinaryvegan.net)
PCRM (pcrm.org)
Plantz St. (plantbasedkatie.com)
Plant Powered Kitchen (plantpoweredkitchen.com)
Potato Strong (potatostrong.com)
Straight Up Food (straightupfood.com)
The Vegan 8 (thevegan8.com)
Vegan Junction (veganjunction.com)

Further Education/Classes
eCornell Nutrition Studies (ecornell.com/certificates/plant-based-nutrition/certificate-in-plant-based-nutrition/)
Forks over Knives Cooking Course by Rouxbe online cooking school (forksoverknives.com/cooking-course/#gs.rxuQzr8)

PCRM and George University free online continuing education credits (nutritioncme.org)

PCRM Food for Life Certification Training (pcrm.org/health/diets/ffl/ffl-the-power-of-food-for-health)

McDougall Starch Solution Certification for Professional and Non-Professionals (drmcdougall.com)

REFERENCES

[1]McDougall, John A., and Mary A. McDougall. *The starch solution: eat the foods you love, regain your health, and lose the weight for good!* New York: Rodale, 2013.

[2]"Obesity in the US Fast Facts." CNN. July 11, 2017. Accessed November 12, 2016. http://www.cnn.com/2013/09/02/health/obesity-in-u-s-fast-facts/.

[3]"National Center for Health Statistics." Centers for Disease Control and Prevention. May 03, 2017. Accessed November 12, 2016. https://www.cdc.gov/nchs/fastats/heart-disease.htm.

[4]Kemmis, Karen, PT, DPT, MS, CDE, FAADE. "American Association of Diabetes Educators." The 2017 National Diabetes Statistics Report is Here. Accessed March 13, 2018. https://www.diabeteseducator.org/news/aade-blog/aade-blog-details/karen-kemmis-pt-dpt-ms-cde-faade/2017/07/26/the-2017-national-diabetes-statistics-report-is-here.

[5]"High Blood Pressure Facts." Centers for Disease Control and Prevention. November 30, 2016. Accessed November 12, 2016. https://www.cdc.gov/bloodpressure/facts.htm.

[6]"Stroke." Centers for Disease Control and Prevention. September 06, 2017. Accessed November 12, 2016. https://www.cdc.gov/stroke/facts.htm.

[7]"Cancer Survivorship." Centers for Disease Control and Prevention. May 30, 2017. Accessed November 12, 2016. https://www.cdc.gov/cancer/survivorship/basic_info/survivors/index.htm.

[8]"Chronic Disease Prevention and Health Promotion." Centers for Disease Control and Prevention. September 12, 2017. Accessed November 12, 2016. https://www.cdc.gov/chronicdisease/resources/publications/aag/alzheimers.htm.

[9]"Osteoporosis fast facts." National Osteoporosis Foundation. Accessed November 12, 2016 from https://cdn.nof.org/wp-content/uploads/2015/12/Osteoporosis-Fast-Facts.pdf

[10]"Facts about Arthritis." Accessed November 12, 2016. http://www.idph.state.il.us/about/womenshealth/factsheets/arthrit.htm.

[11]Campbell, T. Colin. eCornell Certificate in Plant-Based Nutrition Course Diet and Cancer 1. Diseases of affluence, diet and cancer I: Chemical causes of cancer. May 2016.

[12]"Diet: Only Hope for Arthritis." Dr. McDougall's Health & Medical Center. Accessed November 5, 2015. https://www.drmcdougall.com/health/education/health-science/featured-articles/articles/diet-only-hope-for-arthritis/.

[13]Greger, Michael. "What Causes Insulin Resistance?" NutritionFacts.org. January 6, 2017. Accessed January 20, 2017. http://nutritionfacts.org/video/what-causes-insulin-resistance/.

[14]"Alzheimer's Disease." Alzheimer's disease | Health Topics | NutritionFacts.org. December 2, 2016. Accessed December 2, 2016. http://nutritionfacts.org/topics/alzheimers-disease/.

[15]"The Protein Myth." The Physicians Committee. November 15, 2016. Accessed March 13, 2018. http://www.pcrm.org/health/diets/vsk/vegetarian-starter-kit-protein.

[16]Campbell, T. Colin. "Nutrition, Politics, and the Destruction of Scientific Integrity." Center for Nutrition Studies. August 16, 2016. Accessed September 6, 2016. http://nutritionstudies.org/nutrition-politics-and-destruction-of-scientific-integrity/.

[17]McDougall, John A., and Mary A. McDougall. *The starch solution: eat the foods you love, regain your health, and lose the weight for good!* New York: Rodale, 2013.

[18]McDougall, John A., and Mary A. McDougall. *The starch solution: eat the foods you love, regain your health, and lose the weight for good!* New York: Rodale, 2013.

[19]Campbell, T. Colin, and Thomas Campbell, II. *The China study: the most comprehensive study of nurtrition ever conducted and the starling implications for diet, weight loss and long-term health (1st ed).* Dallas, TX.: Benbella Books, 2005.

[20]Oliveira, Rosane. "Should You Eat Rice?" UC Davis Integrative Medicine. August 08, 2016. Accessed August 10, 2016. http://ucdintegrativemedicine.com/2016/08/should-you-eat-rice/#gs.fYW_dBo.

[21] Esselstyn, Caldwell Jr. "Abolishing Heart Disease." Center for Nutrition Studies. Ocober 15, 2013. Accessed January 28, 2017. http://nutritionstudies.org/abolishing-heart-disease/.

[22]Campbell, T. Colin. eCornell Certificate in Plant-Based Nutrition Course One: Nutrition Fundamentals. "An investigation begins: Experimental studies on protein." November 2014.

Campbell, T. Colin, and Thomas Campbell, II. *The China study: the most comprehensive study of nurtrition ever conducted and the starling implications for diet, weight loss and long-term health (1st ed).* Dallas, TX.: Benbella Books, 2005.

[23]McDougall, John A. "When friends ask: Where do you get your protein?" The McDougall Newsletter. Accessed February 9, 2014. http://www.drmcdougall.com/misc/2007nl/apr/protein.htm.

Novick, Jeff. "The Myth of Complementary Protein." Forks Over Knives. April 13, 2016. Accessed January 27, 2017. https://www.forksoverknives.com/the-myth-of-complementary-protein/.

[24]McDougall, John A. "Protein overload." The McDougall Newsletter January 2004 - Protein Overload. Accessed September 23, 2016. https://www.drmcdougall.com/misc/2004nl/040100puproteinoverload.htm.

[25]Song, Mingyang, Teresa Fung, and Frank Hu. "Association of Animal and Plant Protein Intake With All Cause and Cause-Specific Mortality." JAMA Internal Medicine. October 01, 2016. Accessed October 20, 2016. http://archinte.jamanetwork.com/article.aspx?articleid=2540540.

[26] Hagan, Kaitlin, Stephanie E, Stampfer, Meir J, Katz, Jeffrey N, Grodstein, and Francine. "Greater Adherence to the Alternative Healthy Eating Index Is Associated with Lower Incidence of Physical Function Impairment in the Nurses' Health Study | The Journal of Nutrition | Oxford Academic." OUP Academic. May 11, 2016. Accessed April 16, 2017. http://jn.nutrition.org/

content/early/2016/05/11/jn.115.227900.short?rss=1&cited-by= yes&legid=nutrition%3Bjn.115.227900v1.

Shah, Allie. "Snacking on nuts, fruits and veggies can help older women remain active." Star Tribune. July 06, 2016. Accessed July 12, 2016. http://www.startribune.com/snacking-on-nuts-fruits-and-veggies-can-help-older-women-reamain-active/385701861/.

[27]Esselstyn, Caldwell B. *Prevent and reverse heart disease: the revolutionary, scientifically proven, nutrition-based cure.* 1st ed. Paperback. New York, NY: Avery, 2007.

[28]McDougall, John A. "Vegetable Fat as Medicine." Dr. McDougall's Health & Medical Center. Accessed August 3, 2017. https://www.drmcdougall.com/health/education/health-science/featured-articles/articles/vegetable-fat-as-medicine/.

[29]McDougall, John A., and Mary A. McDougall. *The starch solution: eat the foods you love, regain your health, and lose the weight for good!* New York: Rodale, 2012.

[30]McDougall, John A., and Mary A. McDougall. *The starch solution: eat the foods you love, regain your health, and lose the weight for good!* New York: Rodale, 2012.

[31]Mapes, Lynda V. "Drugs found in Puget Sound salmon from tainted wastewater." The Seattle Times. February 23, 2016. Accessed October 31, 2017. https://www.seattletimes.com/seattle-news/environment/drugs-flooding-into-puget-sound-and-its-salmon/.

[32] McDougall, John A., and Mary A. McDougall. *The starch solution: eat the foods you love, regain your health, and lose the weight for good!* New York: Rodale, 2012.

[33] "Webinar: 07/28/16, Dr. Anthony Lim, MD, and "The Secret" to Weight Loss." Dr. McDougall's Health & Medical Center. July 28, 2016. Accessed July 28, 2016. https://www.drmcdougall.com/health/education/webinars/webinar-07-28-16/.

[34] Lilse, Douglas J. and Alan Goldhamer, A. *The pleasure trap: Mastering the hidden force that undermines health & happiness.* Summertown, TN: Healthy Living Publications, 2006.

[35] Lustig, Robert. The Food Revolution Summit, Volume 3. "Sugar: A deadly addiction." 2014.

[36] McDougall, John A. "Depression and Anxiety." Dr. McDougall's Health & Medical Center. Accessed January 30, 2017. https://www.drmcdougall.com/health/education/health-science/common-health-problems/depression-and-anxiety/.

[37] Mujcic, R., and A. Oswald. "Evolution of Well-Being and Happiness After Increases in Consumption of Fruit and Vegetables." American journal of public health. August 2016. Accessed October 12, 2016. https://www.ncbi.nlm.nih.gov/pubmed/27400354.

[38] Williams, Erin. "How My Daughter Got off ADHD Meds, Reversed Prediabetes, and Started Thriving on a WFPB Diet." Forks Over Knives. June 23, 2016. Accessed June 24, 2016. https://www.forksoverknives.com/daughter-got-off-multiple-meds-reversed-prediabetes-started-thriving-wfpb-diet/#gs.2YcOUmY.

Greger, Michael. "Preventing Alzheimer's Disease with Diet." NutritionFacts.org. July 26, 2016. Accessed July 26, 2016. https://nutritionfacts.org/2016/07/26/preventing-alzheimers-disease-diet/.

[39] "Chronic Disease Prevention and Health Promotion | CDC." Centers for Disease Control and Prevention. Accessed December 12, 2016. https://www.cdc.gov/chronicdisease/.

[40] Pear, Robert. "Health Spending in U.S. Topped $3 Trillion Last Year." The New York Times. December 02, 2015. Accessed January 30, 2017. https://www.nytimes.com/2015/12/03/us/politics/health-spending-in-us-topped-3-trillion-last-year.html?_r=0.

[41] "US Health System Ranks Last Among Eleven Countries on Measures of Access, Equity, Quality, Efficiency, and Healthy Lives." The Commonwealth Fund. June 16, 2014. Accessed January 27, 2017. http://www.commonwealthfund.org/publications/press-releases/2014/jun/us-health-system-ranks-last.

[42] "Foodborne Illness." The Physicians Committee for Responsible Medicine. Accessed November 9, 2016. http://www.pcrm.org/health/health-topics/foodborne-illness.

[43] "Foodborne Illness." The Physicians Committee for Responsible Medicine. Accessed November 9, 2016. http://www.pcrm.org/health/health-topics/foodborne-illness.

[44] Tuso, P., M. Ismail, B. Ha, and C. Bartolotto. "Nutritional Update for Physicians: Plant-Based Diets." The Permanente Journal - Kaiser Permanente. Spring 2013. Accessed August 10, 2014. http://www.

thepermanentejournal.org/issues/2013/spring/5117-nutrition.html.

[45] Barron, Robert. Word on Fire Catholic Ministries. "Daily gospel reflection.1st week in ordinary time, year I, Mark 1:29–39." January 11, 2017.

[46] "What is Endometriosis? - Endometriosis Association." Endometriosis Assn. Accessed January 30, 2017. http://www.endometriosisassn.org/endo.html.

[47] "Endometriosis." The Physicians Committee for Responsible Medicine. Accessed January 30, 2017. http://www.pcrm.org/health/health-topics/endometriosis.

[48] Esselstyn, Rip. *My beef with meat: the healthiest argument for eating a plant-strong diet plus 140 new Engine 2 recipes.* 1st ed. New York: Grand Central Life & Style, 2013.

[49] Heidrich, Ruth. "How Not to Need Viagra." Forks Over Knives. June 18, 2014. Accessed January 30, 2017. https://www.forksoverknives.com/how-not-to-need-viagra/.

[50] "Paula: Cured Endometriosis." Dr. McDougall's Health & Medical Center. Accessed November 12, 2016. https://www.drmcdougall.com/health/education/health-science/stars/stars-written/paula/.

[51] "In Vitro Fertilization (IVF): Side Effects and Risks." American Pregnancy Association. July 28, 2017. Accessed July 30, 2017. http://americanpregnancy.org/infertility/in-vitro-fertilization/.

Catechism of the Catholic Church #2377 and #2375 cite Joseph Cardinal Ratzinger, Prefect for the Congregation for the Doctrine of the Faith, *Donum vitae, II, 5 and intro, 2. 1987.*

[52]Greger, Michael. "Meat Hormones & Female Infertility." NutritionFacts.org. November 26, 2009. Accessed August 2, 2016. http://nutritionfacts.org/video/meat-hormones-female-infertility/.

[53]Greger, Michael. "Meat Hormones & Female Infertility." NutritionFacts.org. November 26, 2009. Accessed August 2, 2016. http://nutritionfacts.org/video/meat-hormones-female-infertility/.

[54]Chavarro, Jorge E., Janet W. Rich-Edwards, Bernard A. Rosner, and Walter C. Willett. "Protein intake and ovulatory infertility." American journal of obstetrics and gynecology. February 2008. Accessed May 30, 2016. https://www.ncbi.nlm.nih.gov/pmc/articles/PMC3066040/.

[55]"Paula: Cured Endometriosis." Dr. McDougall's Health & Medical Center. Accessed November 12, 2016. https://www.drmcdougall.com/health/education/health-science/stars/stars-written/paula/.

[56]Greger, Michael. "Maternal Diet May Affect Stress Responses in Children." NutritionFacts.org. August 10, 2016. Accessed August 10, 2016. http://nutritionfacts.org/video/maternal-diet-may-affect-stress-responses-in-children/.

[57]Agarwal, Ulka. "Foods that Fight Depression." The Physicians Committee for Responsible Medicine. February 27, 2015. Accessed November 4, 2016. http://www.pcrm.org/nbBlog/index.php/foods-that-fight-depression.

[58]Rapaport, Lisa. "Vegetarian and vegan diets good for kids and adults, nutritionists say." Reuters. December 01, 2016. Accessed December 24, 2016. https://www.reuters.com/article/us-health-nutrition-vegetarian-vegan/vegetarian-and-vegan-diets-good-for-kids-and-adults-nutritionists-say-idUSKBN13Q5R4.

Associated Press. "Doctors: Babies Can Safely be Raised Vegan." VOA. October 21, 2016. Accessed December 5, 2016. http://www.voanews.com/a/babies-can-safely-be-raised-vegan-doctors-say/3561798.html.

McDougall, John A. "Pregnancy & Children." Dr. McDougall's Health & Medical Center. Accessed December 4, 2016. https://www.drmcdougall.com/health/education/health-science/hot-topics/nutrition-topics/pregnancy-children/.

McDougall, John A. "Diet, children, and the future." McDougall Newsletter: September 2012 - Diet, Children, and the Future. September 2012. Accessed December 10, 2016. https://www.drmcdougall.com/misc/2012nl/sep/children.htm.

[59]"The Academy of Nutrition and Dietetics Publishes Stance on Vegan and Vegetarian Diets." The Physicians Committee for Responsible Medicine. November 29, 2016. Accessed December 10, 2016. http://www.pcrm.org/research/research-news/academy-of-nutrition-and-dietetics-publishes-stance-on-vegan-and-vegetarian-diets.

[60]Greger, Michael. "The Acne-Promoting Effects of Milk." NutritionFacts.org. May 14, 2012. Accessed March 10, 2014. http://nutritionfacts.org/video/the-acne-promoting-effects-of-milk/.

⁶¹Greger, Michael. "The Dietary Link Between Acne & Cancer." NutritionFacts.org. January 7, 2016. Accessed July 1, 2016. https://nutritionfacts.org/2016/01/07/the-dietary-link-between-acne-and-cancer/.

⁶²Nelson, Nina, and Randa Nelson. "How We Cured Our Cystic Acne With One Simple Diet Change." Forks Over Knives. February 6, 2016. Accessed February 6, 2016. https://www.forksoverknives.com/how-we-cured-our-cystic-acne-with-diet/#gs.yXP4DLU.

⁶³McDougall, John A. "Diet induced precocious puberty." Dr. McDougall's Health & Medical Center. Nov. & Dec. 1997. Accessed January 3, 2017. https://www.drmcdougall.com/newsletter/nov_dec97.html

⁶⁴McDougall, John A. "Diet induced precocious puberty." Dr. McDougall's Health & Medical Center. Nov. & Dec. 1997. Accessed January 3, 2017. https://www.drmcdougall.com/newsletter/nov_dec97.html.

⁶⁵McDougall, John A. "Food, sex, and attractiveness part 1: The role of body weight." November 2015. Accessed November 8, 2016. https://www.drmcdougall.com/misc/2015nl/nov/foodandsex.htm

⁶⁶"Hunger Facts | Action Against Hunger. Accessed January 30, 2017. http://www.actionagainsthunger.org/hunger-facts?gclid=Cj0KEQiA5bvEBRCM6vypnc7QgMkBEiQAUZftQMjnnh1yiadwThm-bOG3ET0xeZhAlMk21cw_GiJucR0aArTr8P8HAQ.

⁶⁷Suchetka, Diane. "Americans are consuming more calories than ever: Fighting Fat." Cleveland.com. April 05, 2010. Accessed November 27, 2017. http://www.cleveland.com/fighting-fat/

index.ssf/2010/04/americans_are_consuming_more_calories_than_ever.html

[68]Anderson, K., and K. Kuhn. "The Facts." Cowspiracy. Accessed December 2, 2016. http://www.cowspiracy.com/facts/.

[69]"U.N. chief: Hunger kills 17,000 kids daily." CNN World. November 17, 2009. Accessed January 11, 2017. http://edition.cnn.com/2009/WORLD/europe/11/17/italy.food.summit/.

[70] Anderson, K., and K. Kuhn. "The Facts." Cowspiracy. Accessed December 2, 2016. http://www.cowspiracy.com/facts/.

[71]Brown, A. "From food desert to plantpure oasis!" Naked Food. Winter 2017. Ft. Lauderdale, FL: Naked Republic, Inc.

[72]"Facts on Animal Farming and the Environment." One Green Planet. November 21, 2012. Accessed January 29, 2017. http://www.onegreenplanet.org/animalsandnature/facts-on-animal-farming-and-the-environment/.

[73]Robbins, John. *Diet for a new America: how your food choices affect your health, your happiness, and the future of life on Earth*. Tiburon, CA: H J Kramer, 2012.

[74]"10 Reasons to Say NO to Farmed Animals as 'Gifts'." A Well-Fed World. Accessed March 20, 2016. http://awfw.org/no-animal-gifts/.

[75] Anderson, K., and K. Kuhn. "The Facts." Cowspiracy. Accessed December 2, 2016. http://www.cowspiracy.com/facts/.

[76] "Renewing The Earth." Renewing the Earth. Accessed August 4, 2016. http://www.usccb.org/issues-and-action/human-life-and-dignity/environment/renewing-the-earth.cfm

[77] Pimental, D. "The environmental impact of food production part 1." eCornell Certificate in Plant-Based Nutrition Course. May 2016.

[78] Farber, Madeline. "The U.S. Government Is About To Buy 11 Million Pounds of Cheese." Fortune. August 24, 2016. Accessed January 20, 2017. http://fortune.com/2016/08/24/usda-buy-cheese-surplus/.

Gantz, A. (2016, August 24). USDA to buy surplus eggs, egg products. Accessed January 17, 2017. http://www.wattagnet.com/articles/27989-usda-to-buy-surplus-eggs-egg-products.

[79] "Egg Company Reports $74M Loss Due to Vegan Alternatives." The Daily Berries. November 07, 2017. Accessed November 14, 2017. http://www.thedailyberries.com/egg-company-reports-74m-loss-due-vegan-alternatives/.

[80] Robbins, John. *Diet for a new America: how your food choices affect your health, your happiness, and the future of life on Earth.* Tiburon, CA: H J Kramer, 2012.

[81] "Renewing The Earth." Renewing the Earth. Accessed August 4, 2016. http://www.usccb.org/issues-and-action/human-life-and-dignity/environment/renewing-the-earth.cfm.

[82] "Renewing The Earth." Renewing the Earth. Accessed August 4, 2016. http://www.usccb.org/issues-and-action/human-life-and-dignity/environment/renewing-the-earth.cfm.

[83] Pope Benedict XVI. "Caritas in Veritate." Caritas in veritate (June 29, 2009) | BENEDICT XVI. 2009. Accessed June 15, 2016. http://w2.vatican.va/content/benedict-xvi/en/encyclicals/documents/hf_ben-xvi_enc_20090629_caritas-in-veritate.html.

[84] Pope Francis. *Laudato Si: on care for our common home.* Huntington, IN: Our Sunday Visitor, 2015.

[85] "Tackling Climate Change through Livestock." Fao.org. 2007. Accessed January 17, 2014. http://www.fao.org/ag/againfo/resources/en/publications/tackling_climate_change/index.htm.

[86] Goodland, Robert, and Jeff Anhang. "Livestock and Climate Change." Livestock and Climate Change | Worldwatch Institute. 2009. Accessed July 30, 2016. http://www.worldwatch.org/node/6294.

[87] Anderson, K., and K. Kuhn. "The Facts." Cowspiracy. Accessed December 2, 2016. http://www.cowspiracy.com/facts/.

[88] Anderson, K., and K. Kuhn. "The Facts." Cowspiracy. Accessed December 2, 2016. http://www.cowspiracy.com/facts/.

[89] Anderson, K., and K. Kuhn. "The Facts." Cowspiracy. Accessed December 2, 2016. http://www.cowspiracy.com/facts/.

[90] Tuthill, Samantha-Rae. "Deforestation of Amazon Could Alter Global Weather." Local Weather from AccuWeather.com - SuperiorAccuracy™. November 23, 2013. Accessed December 3, 2016. http://www.accuweather.com/en/weather-news/amazon-climate-change/20184965.

[91] Butler, Rhett A. "Deforestation causes 25% of greenhouse gas emissions." Conservation news. December 10, 2005. Accessed January 31, 2017. https://news.mongabay.com/2005/12/deforestation-causes-25-of-greenhouse-gas-emissions/.

[92] McWilliams, James. "Opinion | Meat Makes the Planet Thirsty." The New York Times. March 7, 2014. Accessed April 7, 2015. http://mobile.nytimes.com/2014/03/08/opinion/meat-makes-the-planet-thirsty.html?_r=0&referrer.

[93] "Factory Farms." A Well-Fed World. Accessed November 2, 2016. http://awfw.org/factory-farms/.

[94] "Pollution | National Wildlife Federation." The National Wildlife Federation. Accessed January 24, 2017. https://www.nwf.org/Educational-Resources/Wildlife-Guide/Threats-to-Wildlife/Pollution.

Monger, B. "Environmental impact of food production II." eCornell Certificate in Plant-Based Nutrition Course. May 2016.

[95] Potera, Carol. "Food safety: US rice serves up arsenic." Environmental Health Perspectives. June 2007. Accessed September 12, 2017. https://www.ncbi.nlm.nih.gov/pmc/articles/PMC1892142/.

[96] Peplow, Mark. "US rice may carry an arsenic burden." Nature News. August 02, 2005. Accessed September 12, 2017. http://www.nature.com/news/2005/050801/full/news050801-5.html.

[97] Greger, Michael. "Cancer Risk from Arsenic in Rice & Seaweed." NutritionFacts.org. July 24, 2017. Accessed September 12, 2017. https://nutritionfacts.org/video/cancer-risk-from-arsenic-in-rice-and-seaweed/?utm_source=NutritionFacts.org&utm_campaign=0cf9cd9183-RSS_VIDEO_DAILY&utm_medium=email&utm_term=0_40f9e497d1-0cf9cd9183-23332677&mc_cid=0cf9cd9183&mc_eid=0aa965a87b.

[98] "Renewing The Earth." Renewing the Earth. Accessed August 4, 2016. http://www.usccb.org/issues-and-action/human-life-and-dignity/environment/renewing-the-earth.cfm.

[99] Robbins, John. *Diet for a new America: how your food choices affect your health, your happiness, and the future of life on Earth*. Tiburon, CA: H J Kramer, 2012.

[100] John Robbins: Julia Child Gave Up Veal (VIDEO) - Vegsource.com. March 1, 2010. Accessed January 29, 2017. http://www.vegsource.com/news/2010/03/john-robbins-julia-child-gave-up-veal-video.html

[101] McWilliams, James. "Spring 2014." The American Scholar. March 11, 2014. Accessed October 13, 2016. https://theamericanscholar.org/issues/spring-2014/.

[102]"Renewing The Earth." Renewing the Earth. Accessed August 4, 2016. http://www.usccb.org/issues-and-action/human-life-and-dignity/environment/renewing-the-earth.cfm.

[103]Eaton, Akisha Townsend. "Pope Francis, Animals and the Season of Creation: A Millennial's Perspective." The Huffington Post. October 02, 2016. Accessed November 19, 2016. http://www.huffingtonpost.com/akisha-townsend-eaton/pope-frances-and-animals_b_8224480.html.

[104]Robbins, John. *Diet for a new America: how your food choices affect your health, your happiness, and the future of life on Earth.* Tiburon, CA: H J Kramer, 2012.

[105]"Slaughterhouse Workers Have PTSD From Killing Animals. Here's Why That Matters..." The Daily Berries. Accessed October 7, 2017. http://www.thedailyberries.com/slaughterhouse-workers-ptsd-killing-animals-heres-matters/.

[106]Greger, Michael. "Can We Fight the Blues with Greens?" NutritionFacts.org. March 27, 2014. Accessed October 30, 2016. http://nutritionfacts.org/2014/03/27/can-we-fight-the-blues-with-greens/.

Beezhold, B. L., and C. S. Johnston. "Restriction of meat, fish, and poultry in omnivores improves mood: a pilot randomized controlled trial." Nutrition journal. February 14, 2012. Accessed January 29, 2017. https://www.ncbi.nlm.nih.gov/pubmed/22333737.

107 Camosy, Charles. "The case for animal welfare as a matter of faith." Crux. August 06, 2016. Accessed August 6, 2016. https://cruxnow.com/church-in-the-usa/2016/08/06/case-animal-welfare-matter-faith/.

108 "New Research Finds Vast Majority of Americans Concerned about Farm Animal Welfare, Confused by Food Labels and Willing to Pay More for Better Treatment." ASPCA. July 7, 2016. Accessed July 12, 2016. http://www.aspca.org/about-us/press-releases/new-research-finds-vast-majority-americans-concerned-about-farm-animal.

109 Longley, Robert. "Up to 75 Percent of US Youth Ineligible for Military Service." ThoughtCo. July 5, 2016. Accessed August 12, 2016. http://usgovinfo.about.com/od/usmilitary/a/unabletoserve.htm.

Suchetka, Diane. "Americans are consuming more calories than ever: Fighting Fat." Cleveland.com. April 05, 2010. Accessed November 27, 2017. http://www.cleveland.com/fighting-fat/index.ssf/2010/04/americans_are_consuming_more_calories_than_ever.html.

110 Roll, Rich. Rich Roll Facebook Page. December 20, 2016. Accessed December 20, 2016. https://www.facebook.com/richrollfans/?fref=ts.

111 Roberts, Holly. *Vegetarian Christian saints: mystics, ascetics & monks*. San Francisco, CA: Anjeli Press, 2004.

[112]Kucinich, Elizabeth. "Say "YES" to organic." *May 31, 2016*. Retrieved January 28, 2017. http://rodaleinstitute.org/say-yes-to-organic/

[113]"Renewing The Earth." Renewing the Earth. Accessed August 4, 2016. http://www.usccb.org/issues-and-action/human-life-and-dignity/environment/renewing-the-earth.cfm.

[114]Greger, Michael. "Where Do You Get Your Fiber?" NutritionFacts.org. September 29, 2015. Accessed September 29, 2015. http://nutritionfacts.org/2015/09/29/where-do-you-get-your-fiber/.

[115]Melina, Vesanto, Craig Winston, and Susan Levin. "Position of the Academy of Nutrition and Dietetics: Vegetarian diets." December 2016. Accessed January 26, 2017. http://www.andjrnl.org/article/S2212-2672(16)31192-3/pdf.

Starostinetskaya, Anna. "Academy of Nutrition and Dietetics Greenlights Veganism." VegNews.com. December 1, 2016. Accessed December 1, 2016. http://vegnews.com/articles/page.do?pageId=8698&catId=1.

[116]McDougall, John A., and Mary A. McDougall. *The starch solution: eat the foods you love, regain your health, and lose the weight for good!* New York: Rodale, 2013.

[117]Greger, Michael. "Which Type of Protein Is Better for Our Kidneys?" NutritionFacts.org. October 30, 2015. Accessed September 19, 2016. http://www.nutritionfacts.org/video/which-type-of-protein-is-better-for-our-kidneys/.

[118]Campbell, T. Colin, and Thomas Campbell, II. *The China study: the most comprehensive study of nurtrition ever conducted and the starling implications for diet, weight loss and long-term health (1st ed).* Dallas, TX.: Benbella Books, 2005.

[119]Campbell, T. Colin. eCornell Certificate in Plant-Based Nutrition Course. "Nutrient fundamentals II: An overemphasis on protein." 2014.

[120]Kristensen, M. D., N. T. Bendsen, S. M. Christensen, A. Astrup, and A. Raben. "Meals based on vegetable protein sources (beans and peas) are more satiating than meals based on animal protein sources (veal and pork) - a randomized cross-over meal test study." Food & nutrition research. October 19, 2016. Accessed January 4, 2017. https://www.ncbi.nlm.nih.gov/pubmed/27765144.

[121]Klaper, Michael. "Vegan Protein Deficiency." Michael Klaper, M.D., Nutrition-Based Medicine. Accessed September 10, 2016. http://doctorklaper.com/videos/vegan-protein-deficiency/.

Pineda Ochoa, Sofia. "Vitamin B12: All Your Questions Answered." Forks Over Knives. November 16, 2017. Accessed December 5, 2017. https://www.forksoverknives.com/vitamin-b12-questions-answered-2/#gs.VvZw8uA.

[122]Barnard, Neal. "Ask Dr. Neal Barnard: Do I need vitamin B12?" YouTube. December 19, 2013. Accessed July 12, 2016. https://www.youtube.com/watch?v=QyTjS80Dyk0.

[123]Campbell, T. Colin, and Howard Jacobson. *Whole: rethinking the science of nutrition.* Dallas: Benbella Books, 2013.

¹²⁴"World health org and UN recommend populations eat plant-based diet." Vegsource.com. May 16, 2010. Accessed January 31, 2017. http://www.vegsource.com/news/2010/05/world-health-org-and-un-recommend-populations-eat-plant-based-diets.html.

¹²⁵Kirchgaessner, Stephanie. "Five Star mayor of Turin to create Italy's first 'vegetarian city'." The Guardian. July 21, 2016. Accessed August 2, 2016. https://www.theguardian.com/world/2016/jul/21/turin-mayor-italys-first-vegetarian-city-five-star.

¹²⁶Starostinetskaya, Anna. "Ireland's Former President Urges Young Leaders to Go Vegan." VegNews.com. September 30, 2016. Accessed September 30, 2016. http://vegnews.com/articles/page.do?pageId=8440&catId=1.

¹²⁷Starostinetskaya, Anna. "New Zealand's First Vegan Governor General Sworn In." VegNews.com. October 3, 2016. Accessed October 3, 2016. http://vegnews.com/articles/page.do?ageId=8449&catId=1.

¹²⁸Campbell, T. Colin, and Thomas Campbell, II. *The China study: the most comprehensive study of nurtrition ever conducted and the starling implications for diet, weight loss and long-term health (1ˢᵗ ed)*. Dallas, TX.: Benbella Books, 2005.

¹²⁹Milman, Oliver, and Stuart Leavenworth. "China's plan to cut meat consumption by 50% cheered by climate campaigners." The Guardian. June 20, 2016. Accessed July 18, 2016. https://www.theguardian.com/world/2016/jun/20/chinas-meat-consumption-climate-change.

[130]Simon, David Robinson. "10 Things We Wish Everyone Knew About the Meat and Dairy Industries." PETA. Accessed January 30, 2017. http://www.peta.org/living/food/10-things-wish-everyone-knew-meat-dairy-industries/.

[131]Greger, Michael. "Evidence-Based Eating." NutritionFacts.org. January 4, 2017. Accessed January 4, 2017. http://nutritionfacts.org/video/evidence-based-eating/?utm_source=NutritionFacts.org&utm_campaign=3556740102-RSS_VIDEO_DAILY&utm_medium=email&utm_term=0_40f9e497d1-3556740102-23332677&mc_cid=3556740102&mc_eid=918ec707c1.

[132]Associated Press. "Doctors: Babies Can Safely be Raised Vegan." VOA. October 21, 2016. Accessed December 5, 2016. http://www.voanews.com/a/babies-can-safely-be-raised-vegan-doctors-say/3561798.html.

[133]Mirkin, Gabe. "Pesticides." Dr. Gabe Mirkin on Health, Fitness and Nutrition. | Pesticides. January 28, 2017. Accessed January 28, 2017. http://www.drmirkin.com/nutrition/pesticides.html.

[134]Sciammacco, Sara. "More Scientific Evidence That Organic Food Is More Nutritious." EWG. July 15, 2014. Accessed June 21, 2015. http://www.ewg.org/release/more-scientific-evidence-organic-food-more-nutritious.

[135]Mirkin, Gabe. "Saturated Fats from Plants Increase Fat in Liver." Dr. Gabe Mirkin on Health, Fitness and Nutrition. | Saturated Fats from Plants Increase Fat in Liver. March 2, 2014. Accessed March 5, 2014. http://drmirkin.com/nutrition/saturated-fats-from-plants-increase-fat-in-liver.html.

[136] McDougall, John A. "Webinar: 10/29/15, Breast Cancer and The Secret that the Health Industry Doesn't Want You to Know." Dr. McDougall's Health & Medical Center. October 29, 2015. Accessed November 5, 2015. https://www.drmcdougall.com/health/education/webinars/webinar-10-29-15/.

[137] "The Threats of Overfishing: Consequences at the Commercial Level." DUJS Online. March 11, 2012. Accessed October 31, 2017. http://dujs.dartmouth.edu/2012/03/the-threats-of-overfishing-consequences-at-the-commercial-level/#.Wfi3OHZrxLM.

Made in the USA
Middletown, DE
30 November 2018